Get Balanced
The Natural Way to Better Health
with Superfoods

Written by
Jan Lovejoy

To re-order: call 1 (866) 599-7022

For information or order inquiries, contact:
SGN Nutrition, LLC.
2225 Faraday Ave. Suite E
Carlsbad, CA. 92008

Published by SGN Nutrition, LLC.

Printed in the United States of America

ISBN# 978-0-9791803-0-9

Dedication

· ·

PATTI CANASTRO

My beloved friend and mentor who blessed me with her zest for life and spirit of adventure. My life is richer because she lived.

By the shinning beach of Newport
In a time now long remembered
Stood a tiny house that sheltered a young Mr. and his wife.
And this mister fished the waters,
Knew their power and their splendor
And his Mrs. loved the laughing dancing waves that gave her life.
So their kinship with the ocean spawned a precious child of beauty
Who was formed of sea and sunlight
And whose eyes shone like the waters
When they turn from green to blue.
As a baby she would listen to the wind-songs of the mermaids
Who would tell of far off islands and the mysteries of the sea.
As a girl she gathered sea shells
That would whisper of the wonders
To be found by those who ventured on the pathways of the deep.
All those days she yearned and listened
For a voice that would direct her
To the golden isle of promise
Where her heart so longed to be.
Many years her soul would wander
Many nights her mind would ponder
How to reach the place of yonder
Where her spirit would find 'home'.
She would hold tight all the treasures
That the earth so gladly gave her
She would store up all the beauty
In the hope-chest of her heart.
When she found her life's companion,
They set sail for moon-lit canyons
To explore the emerald valleys and the sparkling sapphire sea.
As the years swept by like tall ships
Gently sailing ever-onward,
As her children bore their children
And her life on earth was blessed.
All her dreams turned into hours and the hours turned to riches
All the pennies turned to dollars
And the laughter became rest.

She would muse upon the meaning
Of the treasures she had gathered,
All the love, that had, like driftwood
Been made smoother by the storms.
Now she knew that home was more than
What's been formed by some volcano
What's been hammered bought or grown.
Home's a candle that, when once lit,
In the hearts of all beloved
Can never be extinguished… and never really owned.
But when one heart finds safe harbor
In the outstretched arms of others,
There are signal fires in heaven
Lit by love's unchanging hand.
So when the great flame turned to embers
In the fire of her journey,
She surrendered all her cargo
To a ship no one can see.
When her hands released their holding
And her eyes ceased their beholding
Love herself enfolded
In a gold and graceful sea.
So from hoping and imagining
To a world of ever-knowing,
She's at home in love more loving
And more free than we believe.
In an eternity much longer,
In a joy that is far stronger,
In a place where life's much deeper
And much wider than the sea.
So when we hear the lilting chant
Of waves upon the beach,
We'll raise our glass to one
Whose gentle strength our souls did teach,
Whose courageous heart
Our hearts did reach.

By Claudia Lovejoy

Acknowledgments

. . . .

ANTHONY MISNER: Your endless courage has given me the confidence to go forward with this book and with our business. What a blessing you have been these past 33 years! In giving birth to you, I gave birth to the best part of myself.

ROSE CRIMMEY: You are a treasured friend whose passion for health and love for me has been an inspiration to my work and a light upon my path.

CLAUDIA LOVEJOY: Thank you for introducing me to the glory of God and praying for me as I learned to walk in the Spirit.

TOM PURDY: Remember stalking the wild mushroom together in the shady forests of the Northwest? Little did we know that those humbling beginnings would open the door to the healing wonders of God's amazing garden. Best friends are friends to the end!

ABEL VALLS: My dearest friend who has encouraged me in every possible way and helped me to communicate the deep truths that once were silent within me.

VICKI COMER & RANDEE COFFMAN: You are more than sisters; you are my dearly cherished friends. For the past five decades, you have known me, loved me, cried with me, laughed with me and believed in me through every step of my life's journey.

DAD & MOM: You have been, and always will be, my heroes. Your amazing personalities, incredible parenting and relentless commitment to each other gave me a great passion for life. When you taught me how to laugh at the ups and downs of human existence, you gave me the greatest gift of all: a balanced perspective and a happy heart.

CLEGG HUBBELL & BRIAN RAMSEIER: You guys faithfully ran interference for days, weeks and months while I typed away at this book. Without you, SGN Nutrition might never have become a reality…let alone a success!

DONNA MOORE: A superwoman who skillfully helped to birth this book on superfoods.

And to all those who have encouraged me and believed in me, but too numerous to mention, thank you.

Table Of Contents

Foreword

For eons early man has struggled to survive. Survival depended upon the ability to endure through long periods of inadequate food supply. Consequently most evolutionary biologists believe we have a gene(s) that aided the survival potential for man. This gene(s) is believed to have performed two very interesting functions. One function was the capability of hunters to store fat as an instant energy source to survive lean times. The second feature of this inheritance dealt with the metabolic ability to shift the body's metabolism into fat storage, and preserve as much as possible from the inadequate dietary intake.

For most of today's society the scarcity of food is not as critical as it was in caveman's times. Today, especially in America, there is more than an adequate food supply. All one has to do is to read the headlines, and the emergence of an unhealthy and obese population is being considered as a major threat to the longevity of this and future generations. The same "good" gene(s) that enabled the species to survive, are now operating to the *detriment* of the population in the presence of a more than adequate food supply.

About two decades ago, a small group of scientists reported the concept of immunosenescence, this concept dealt with the aging of the immune system. They proposed that this weakening was responsible for the increased incidence of cancer, cardiovascular disease, and arthritis in the elderly. Their work was defined even further by controlled animal studies where they restricted the caloric intake of laboratory animals. They confirmed their views, but were also surprised to learn that the life spans of these animals increased some 50 to 100%, when the laboratory animals were forced to eat less.

The take-away message from these two observations is that our society is eating too much, resulting in increases in disease, and shortened life spans. One of the interesting theories today which links several diseases together involves the description of something called "Metabolic Syndrome" or "Syndrome X." This new view of disease patterns has coupled diabetes, cardiovascular disease and high blood pressure, high lipids, such as cholesterol and triglyc-erides, obesity, and perhaps cancer. Several investigators have proposed genetic control of these disease states, and it may turn out that these genes may in fact be related to those survival genes about which we spoke earlier. They may "kick in" when food supplies are abundant.

There is then a "double whammy" to the above observations. Too many calories, cause the pathologies associated with Metabolic Syndrome and at the same time begin to wear down the immune system raising our susceptibility to debilitating diseases for the rest of our lives. The pharmaceutical industry is busy conducting inten-sive research looking for compounds that, for example, will control weight, lower cholesterol, control blood pressure, and treat diabetic patients. Interestingly, these same pharmaceutical companies previously looked at all of these symptoms as individual diseases, and developed drugs to treat each of these separately. Now they are finding, that the current drugs for example, that lower cholesterol, sometimes elevate triglycerides; drugs that treat blood pressure, sometimes cause patients to alter their lipids and cause weight gain; drugs that are used to treat diabetes can also cause patients to gain weight, affect blood pressure and lipid profiles.

Perhaps lying at the heart of this modern complexity of life style, overabundance of food, and early disease manifestation may be one important biochemical event, and that is the formation of free radi-cals. These small entities are mostly byproducts of the various biochemical reactions that are taking place in our bodies continually. Obviously the more food we eat, and the more metabolism taking place, the greater the rate of the formation of these free radicals. A considerable body of evidence is indicating that these free radicals have been implicated in almost every pathological condition studied. It is beginning to appear that cancer, arthritis, diabetes, obesity, cardiovascular disease, etc. may have a strong dependence upon the presence of free radicals. Well what does all of this have to do with this book you are about to read. The trends that were discussed point to the individual having the control of his or her own destiny.

The real impact of this book should help you change your lifestyle and especially your eating habits. Not only that, but it will also tell you *why* you want to eat these foods. It gives you the science, written in "plain language" underlying its recommendations, so that you know why the particular food is listed.

Aside from maintaining a regular exercise regiment, the two important themes that you will find in this book is to eat the right foods of course, and thus limit your caloric intake, and to maintain an optimal level of anti-oxidants to help control those nasty free radicals that are circulating through your body waiting to cause and/or exacerbate pathology.

I guarantee that you will not find a more compact nutritional reference guide on superfoods. This book is truly a compendium of nutritional facts and data and will be used not only in meal planning but to understand better what enters our bodies. This book will help us all in understanding how to better adjust our eating habits leading to an overall healthy lifestyle.

Dan Tripodi, PhD, Executive Director
The Sage Group, Branchberg, New Jersey
And Adjunct Professor Biological Sciences,
University of Delaware

Introduction

Get Balanced

The Natural Way to Better Health with Superfoods

Has someone ever walked by and something in your brain automatically spelled out (in big neon letters) the word "HEALTH!"? I'm not talking about beauty here; I'm talking about radiant health, even in middle or old age. Why do some of us have it and some of us don't? Youth and genetics can cut you a lot of slack in your 20s and 30s, but over a lifetime, what you choose to eat will slowly sculpt your entire being. For some of us, that's bad news, but here's the good news: the body has an incredible capacity to heal itself, and it's just waiting for you to start feeding it the nutritional tools necessary for transformation. How do I know this? I'm a walking talking testimony to the power of nutritional healing.

My Story

I was a normal healthy San Diego surfer girl until one fateful day back in 1971 when I got married and started taking birth control pills. In retrospect, I think I would have been better off drinking a lysol-cyanide smoothie, but what 19-year-old suspects such drastic effects from such a popular little pill? It wasn't long before my entire body turned into an allergic nuclear reactor, and when I did become pregnant, I quickly developed an allergy to the very hormones my body had started to produce! Being allergic to yourself is a traumatic experience (to put it mildly), and I continued to suffer physically until the day after I gave birth to my son Anthony. Little did I know, as I happily celebrated Anthony's birth and my liberation from nine months of hormone poisoning, that my problems were just beginning.

Because I continued to struggle with an onslaught of female problems, I was advised that a hysterectomy was a viable option. I was only 25 years old. Although hopeful that this surgery would eliminate my problems, I soon discovered that I was allergic to the hormones my body produced while ovulating, so I went back to the operating table at 32 and had both ovaries removed.

Being more than a little frightened because of my unending health problems, I picked up a copy of *Let's Eat Right To Keep Fit*, written by Adelle Davis in the 1970s. There wasn't much being written about nutrition in those days, but that book opened my eyes to the healing properties found in vitamins and minerals.

I knew that modern medicine wasn't able to provide all the help I needed, so with this little book as my guide, I began to create my own nutritional program to survive the minefield of medically-induced menopause.

Despite all the physical trauma I was experiencing, I managed to move to the Hawaiian island of Kauai in my mid-20s, open a small yardage store and raise my son as a single mom. My subsequent careers as a small business owner, cosmetologist and restaurateur taught me much, but as I entered my 40s, this passionate interest in nutrition led me into my most fulfilling work as an herbalist and formulator of natural food supplements. Although I view every decade of my life as rewarding, I believe my greatest contribution is still ahead as I travel and teach this natural way to health.

Although we live in an age chock-full of medical marvels and miraculous technology, I have listened to literally hundreds of stories similar to my own. So many people in America are sick, and like Humpty-Dumpty, all of their procedures and all of their pills can't put them back together again.

I wholeheartedly support many of the amazing innovations developed by modern medicine, yet I believe these must be knowledgeably combined with the ancient wisdom of alternative medicine. My desire is to share with you, through the reading of this book, the nutritional tools necessary for the healing of your body. Just as I believe that balanced nutrition is a foundation for good health, I also believe that unbalanced nutrition is a foundation for sickness and disease. Making simple changes in how you eat, how you drink and how you move can determine whether you spend your time enjoying life or spend your life trying to buy yourself more time.

What is a Superfood?

Remember that old TV show "MacGyver?" That guy could take regular household items, combine them with his vast supply of scientific knowledge and accomplish just about anything. He could diffuse a nuclear missile with a simple

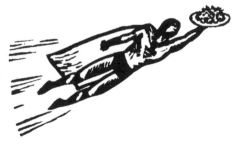

paper clip, or even ignite a homemade bomb with the contents of a cold capsule. His feats were nothing short of amazing, but do you realize that your body is even more creative than MacGyver? The very body that you often neglect uses the lycopene from an ordinary tomato to prevent cancer, extracts the ellagic acid from a walnut to fuel the function of your brain and uses the oleic acid from an olive to strengthen your immune system. These three foods are just a few of the items we now call "Superfoods," ancient but simple sources of nutrition. No one has yet improved on the recipe for fruits, nuts, vegetables and grains, so try as we might, we can't improve or disprove the superiority of Superfoods.

Although we can't improve Superfoods, we can ignore them, and that's been the downfall of modern society. We have opted for the sweeter, saltier, fatter, faster and flashier foods so tempting to the taste buds and so technicolor to the eye. Don't you think it's time to reacquaint ourselves with the food that has sustained mankind for thousands of years, and start eating to live rather than dining to die?

You might call this book "Dick and Jane Discover Superfoods," because in it I've included some very basic information (in alphabetical order, of course). I tell you why these foods are nutritionally important, explain how they work, tell you where to get them, educate you on the quantities you need to eat, offer some recipes and include simple tips for preparation. Finally, I've added some scientific research facts and a technical glossary (for those of you who are less like Dick and Jane and more like MacGyver).

Experience tells me that most people will gravitate towards the chapter pertaining to their particular health issue, and that's just fine. Feel free to skip around from chapter to chapter, but I hope you'll eventually read the whole book. This is life-giving information so I'd recommend keeping it around as a reference. After reading this book, a friend of mine started tucking a copy into her purse and referring to it while walking down the produce aisle. I like that idea! After a few months, I hope the pages of your book are dog-eared and colorfully marked by a wandering blueberry or a juicy tomato!

My Mom

While I was living in Seattle, my sister called to ask if I would consider moving back to California to help care for my mother. After a 55-year marriage to my father, she was now a widow whose health was beginning to deteriorate. Following the diagnoses and treatment of breast cancer, she was having terrible side effects from the drug Tamoxifen. Because of frequent memory lapses, fatigue and even a decrease in her ability to communicate, the doctor decided to take Mom off her medication. But this wasn't the only problem. Although my mother had always been a healthy eater, she was just too tired to prepare meals for herself, and consequently her health was slowly getting worse. Unfortunately, many older people have stopped cooking for themselves (actually, many young people are in the very same boat!) so crackers, cheese, cereal, canned soups and pack-aged foods have become their staple diet.

As I considered how to help my Mom regain her strength, I started thinking about a Superfood that could safely strengthen her health and immune system. I knew she would rather drink a supplement than take another pill, but as an herbalist and nutritionist, I also knew there were certain herbs which would not be advisable for someone on heart medication or cholesterol-lowering drugs. So with all these things in mind, I began to formulate a healthy drink that would taste good (because I knew my Mom wouldn't consider drinking some-thing that tasted like seaweed and yeast!).

I bought a house just a few doors down from Mom, which was a good thing because I had to run ten 100-yard-dashes down that street in the next few months! Her health seemed to be in freefall, and we'd barely get one medical problem taken care of before another would take its place. My mother's heartbeat was becoming erratic, but every time we drove to the hospital, the doctors were not able to find the problem.

She was actually suffering from heart failure and her heart was flickering like a light bulb that was getting ready to go out. Nothing was showing up on the tests, Mom's memory was failing, her ability to walk was impaired and she was becoming increasingly frightened. As her condition worsened one Mother's Day morning, I raced her to the hospital once more, but this time I arrived armed with pages of notes about her symptoms and her blood pressure readings from the previous week. I insisted that something be done to help my Mom, and so the next day they sent her to surgery to receive a pacemaker.

However the pacemaker wasn't the only change necessary. Mom had been lacking the proper nutrients to nourish her blood, brain and heart, so in addition to the Superfood drink, we had Mom eat five small meals a day to help stabilize her blood sugar levels and combat indigestion and fatigue. I am elated to report that she has overcome a "pre-diabetic" condition by changing her diet at 79 years of age! Mom is not only healthier and happier, but has become the designated driver for all of her friends whenever they go out shopping!

I have taught my Mom all about Superfoods, which she has integrated into her lifestyle along with a few supplements. My mom's health has made a complete turnaround, and she's once again able to enjoy her golden years. She's healthy, vibrant, active and the best-looking 80-year-old in San Diego!

My Sister

A few days ago my sister and I piled into the car and headed for the grocery store to buy ingredients for a special birthday dinner. As kids, teenagers and even as young mothers, we probably would have headed straight for the bakery section and "oohed" and "aaahed" over the white cakes covered with blue frosting. But this time our "oohs" and "aaahs" were coming from the produce section! We were acting like kids in a candy store, scooping up bright orange carrots, dandelion greens, baby arugula and fresh bunches of beets. The people around us must have been thinking, "Why are these two 50-something women getting so excited about vegetables?" How did our tastes so drastically change from fried chicken, mashed potatoes, and frosted cake to organic chicken, roasted vegetables and baby greens? As I looked at my once chubby but now radiant sister, all I could think was, "We've come a long way, baby!"

I had to laugh when the checker asked if we were buying the greens for our rabbits at home. "Nope," I exclaimed proudly, "we're making a special dinner for my sister's 57th birthday. Have you ever tried dandelion greens? They're loaded with nutrients and they taste great. I'll give you a hint on how to fix them." After sharing the Gospel of Greens with yet another malnourished matron, we happily strolled to the car with a bounce in our step more common for ladies half our age.

Truth be told, we weren't always like this, but my sister and I have slowly regained our health and vitality by changing our diet, exercise and belief systems. We actually feel better in our mid-fifties than we felt in our mid-thirties (but that's a whole other book!). To quote Bob Dylan: "We were so much older then...we're younger then that now."

My sister, Vicki, has lost 90 pounds over the last five years, 25 of the pounds were lost in the last year. One of the many things I admire about Vicki is her incredible determination to stick with her healthy lifestyle plan. At the beginning, she would put an outfit on a wall in her bedroom, and it was her target outfit. She began to inquire about which foods would give her the nutrient value she needed and would satisfy her need to eat good, healthy, crunchy foods. Vicki wasn't a big eater; her metabolism was just more sluggish than others. Interestingly, she craved hot foods like cayenne pepper and spicy foods (foods that raise the body's metabolism) and found that eating five small meals a day helped maintain a faster more efficient metabolism. Another part of the weight loss puzzle: she visualized herself thinner. She never cursed her body, she just wanted to be healthier and have more energy.

As she ingested Superfoods rich in nutrients, she gradually stopped craving all those "empty calories," And she also started feeling something she hadn't felt for years: ENERGY. Little by little, her body began steering her in a new direction by giving her cravings for the foods that were giving her life. She also found that this new way of eating helped lessen many of the symptoms associated with the medical condition of irritable bowel syndrome (IBS). The desire to eat "comfort foods" to calm herself down has now changed to eating Superfoods to make her energy soar! And because she's gradually become a "water junkie," we tease my sister about the water bottle that's eternally in her hand, day and night. I think the only time she puts that bottle down is when she swims her daily laps in the pool!

My Son

Let me tell you a little bit about my amazing son, Anthony. He is brilliant, energetic, committed, hard-working and capable of accomplishing any goal. By his mid-20s, he was already zooming up the corporate ladder in the hotel business, financially successful and highly-favored by his company. He was running the typical hotel marathon: eating rich food, drinking expensive wine, working too many hours, staying up too late, not getting enough exercise, retaining water, slowing his metabolism, gaining weight and becoming increasingly tired. Why was my young, smart son starting to be forgetful? Why was this even-tempered young man starting to lose his temper?

One day Anthony confessed to me that he'd recently been to the hospital three times because his face was consistently swelling and breaking out in hives. The doctors had no diagnosis for his condition and sent him home with some Benadryl, a powerful antihistamine to counteract allergic reactions. This might have been a good way to reduce his symptoms, but I knew that Benedryl could not heal his body. When I asked if he would be willing to treat his health problems naturally, Anthony immediately said "Yes."

I soon realized that Anthony wasn't getting the nutrients he needed to keep his overworked body in balance. Because his stress level was usually off-the-chart, his body was being continually depleted of valuable B vitamins. He wasn't drinking enough water, so his body was retaining water in order to survive. He was eating quick-fix carbohydrates in order to feed his tired brain, yet he wasn't giving his body the nutrients it so desperately needed. Because his immune system was weakened, Anthony was often sick with sinus infections, colds and flus passed on by all the international travelers coming in and out of the hotel.

Enter Doctor Mom, armed with Superfoods, a high-potency B-Complex vitamin, a container of my superfood drink and a prescription to ride, ride, ride the wild surf whenever he could slip out of the fast lane for a few hours.

Here's the good news: Anthony is now out of the hotel business! And here's the best news: he's now a devoted fan of Superfoods, has a higher metabolism than Speedy Gonzalez and has enough energy to run our company, surf every day, think corporate thoughts and once again enjoy the vitality of youth. What more could a mother want?

As you can tell, my family should all star in a sit-com called "The Balanced Bunch." I have to admit that we're hooked on feeling good, because we've all learned that balancing is not an act. It's a reality that can change your life.

Tom's Story

Many of us have a significant other that we want to help get healthy, I'm no exception. Tom is my friend and former husband who has taken the steps to change his life in all aspects, body, mind and spirit. When I asked him if he would like to contribute his story to the book, he wholeheartedly agreed.

Tom's onset of age related problems began at 47. He had tried to donate blood, but the Blood Bank refused to take it because of high blood pressure. He was shocked to hear that it was 160/110! Blood tests also revealed high cholesterol and triglyceride levels. A diuretic was prescribed for blood pressure and statins for cholesterol; they worked fairly well, although there were side effects. The doctor had been blunt: Change your eating habits and start regular exercise or face a shortened life. Tom admitted he started and stopped so many times he couldn't remember the number. The foods he liked were too tempting and a good test simply gave him license to eat them again. Exercise was boring to him, so consequently he didn't keep it up for very long. His weight stayed 210 to 215 on his 5' 8" frame. One attempt resulted in a weight loss of 20 pounds and excellent test numbers, but soon he reverted to indulging in bad foods and quit exercising again.

About nine years after his initial diagnosis, he made the decision to assault all the problem areas at one time. Although Tom was true to his supplemental program of my superfood drink, omega-3 fish oils, CoQ10, lecithin and a B Complex, he knew he needed to do more. He began shopping for and preparing healthy Superfoods, eating at home and bringing his food to work 95% of the time. His next step was incorporating exercise with weights and a resistance machine that he bought cheaply from someone else who had given up! He then made the most important investment in his life. Instead of working a full time job he decided to work part time and put all his energy into his health. In addition to exercise and nutrition, he sought a compatible church and a skilled mental health therapist. The three-pronged attack worked! He has lost 40 pounds, is stronger, clear headed and the persistent negativity that dogged his life has evapo-rated.

It is fair to note that not everyone can take the time away from a career to do what Tom did. It was an investment most people can't afford. A modified version may be better for someone else, and his spiritual path could well be different from one other people will pursue. Therapy can be a difficult choice, but he was determined to deal with any underlying issues as well. In his own words Tom says, "I realized that I needed to look at all three areas simultaneously to effect change. The main lesson is: Don't give up! The gift of health and vigor is one you will never regret giving yourself."

Summary

Balancing what we eat is easy if we know how to make good nutritional choices. Your food choices have a major impact on your health and insure a more energetic life. *Get Balanced: The Natural Way to Better Health with Superfoods* is a guide to choosing those Superfoods that will put you back on track. You'll learn how to eat Superfoods that impact brain power, and learn which heart healthy Superfoods can contribute to changing cholesterol numbers. The book is full of tips and important information about how to maximize your health. This book has something for everyone, whether you are in great shape, have minor or major health problems or know someone who is unable to get control of their health. *Get Balanced* will provide the first step towards a healthy lifestyle change...so turn the page to begin your journey to a healthier lifestyle!

Chapter 1

. . . .

Superfoods That Promote Brain Function

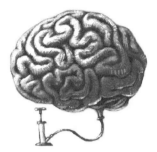

Your brain is the most complex organ in your body, but it's easy to understand its needs. The key is to feed your brain, just like you feed your body. In fact, studies of school kids confirm that the better they eat, the better they learn. Perhaps right next to the bumper sticker that says "My child is an honor student" should be one that says, "If you wanna be below average, eat junk food!" So take a good, hard look at that sugar-laden donut you're getting ready to inhale. It's no surprise that it won't do much to raise your IQ! Then think about how many people will chase that delight with a diet soda in an effort to keep their calories down. Sound familiar?

Your brain needs good, quality foods to give you good, quality mental processes, memory and cognitive abilities. If you're feeling intimi- dated by the thought of game night, it might just be that a steady consumption of Superfoods will increase your brain power **and** your self-confidence.

Brain Bits

✓ Neurons (cells that send and receive electro-chemical signals to and from the brain and nervous system) can send signals to thousands of other neurons at a speed of about 200 miles per hour. There are about 100 billion neurons in the brain.

✓ Chronic stress robs you of brain power. It literally *shrinks and destroys* the brain regions that are crucial for memory.

✓ Your brain can go without oxygen for only 3 to 5 minutes before injury will occur.

✓ Scientists aren't sure how many brain cells you lose each day because of decay and misuse, but no need to worry; you have enough to last for a lifetime!

✓ Unlike cut or scraped skin, or torn and broken bones that mend, your brain cannot repair itself.

✓ Although the brain is only 2% of the body's weight, it uses 20% of the oxygen supply and gets 20% of the blood flow.

✓ Researchers have found a link between the TV viewing habits of elderly individuals and brain power. The more soap operas and TV talk shows they watched, the lower their mental capacity and cognitive skills.

✓ Contrary to old beliefs, we do use all of our brain–not just a small part as previously thought.

✓ The Mozart Effect: listening to a Mozart sonata (or other complex music) can temporarily increase IQ by eight points.

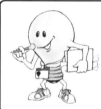 *Quick Tip:* There are several factors causing our accelerated mental decline. Our stressful lives are filled with on-the-go meals consisting of fast food, largely devoid of nutritional value. The result: blood vessels which supply oxygen to the brain get clogged from the side effects of junk food, specifically trans fats and toxins, which reduce the brain's oxygen and nutrient supply.

Superfoods for Brain Function

Blueberries

Why: Packed with antioxidant phytonutrients called anthocyanidins, blueberries neutralize free radical damage to the collagen matrix of cells and tissues. Anthocyanins, the blue-red pigments found in blueberries, actually improve the integrity of veins and vascular system, that means your brain too! Blueberries also enhance the effects of vitamin C. Researchers also have found that blueberries help protect the brain from oxidative stress and may reduce the effects of age-related conditions such as Alzheimer's disease or dementia.

Where to buy it: At grocery stores in the fresh produce section during season (summer) or you can find frozen blueberries year around. If you buy frozen, look for the ones with no sugar added.

How much to take: A ½ cup counts as one of the daily recommended 8 to 10 servings of fruits or vegetables.

> *Quick Facts:* In a study published in the May 2005 issue of the *Journal of Experimental Neurology* it was found that eating blueberries may significantly lessen brain damage from strokes and other neurological disorders.

Lecithin

Why: Lecithin is found in every living cell. Its highest concentrations are in the brain, heart, liver and kidneys. In the brain, lecithin choline is transformed into acetylcholine-needed for transmission of messages from one nerve to another. It's also shown to stimulate the memory. Lecithin's nutrient, phosphatidylcholine, actually nourishes the myelin sheaths surrounding neurons in the brain (the myelin sheath increases transmission speeds of the neurons in the brain) Lecithin is also the emulsifier that keeps fats and cholesterol from clumping together in the blood.

Where to buy it: Health food stores carry it in either granules or capsules. Buy the form most appealing to you.

How much to take: Lecithin is a food, so taking 15 grams a day is perfectly safe. Many people like to eat the granules directly from the container; just chew it up like any other food.

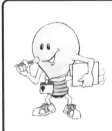

Quick Tip 1: Mix lecithin with a green drink, some flax seed meal and soy protein powder for a fantastic "brain cocktail."
Quick Tip 2: Cooking lecithin does not cause any loss of nutritional value. Lecithin improves the workability of batter or baking mixture and improves the quality of the finished product. You can add lecithin granules to any oil salad dressing for added brain nutrients.
Quick Tip 3: If you are an older person (over 70) or have a cholesterol problem, you might want to increase your lecithin intake to 20 grams daily.

Omega-3 Enriched Eggs

Why: Omega-3 enriched eggs come from hens fed a special diet containing 10–20% ground flaxseed. These eggs are the same as the traditional eggs except they have higher levels of polyunsaturated fatty acid called omega-3 (important for brain function). Eggs are one of nature's most nutrient-dense Superfoods and are one of our richest sources of choline, important for memory. They are high in protein, and one egg contains a relatively high amount of the amino acid tyrosine (for brain power). This Superfood also contains vitamin E, all the B vitamins (including B12, folic acid, niacin) and, in relation to volume, they offer a good supply of calcium.

Where to buy it: Some grocery stores carry these Superfood eggs, but if you can't find them there, visit a health food store.

How much to eat: Eat one omega-3 enriched egg daily or at least four to five enriched eggs weekly.

Sardines

Why: A rich source of DHA (the primary structural component of brain tissue) and other essential fatty acids (EFAs), plus it has a significant amount of DMAE (a powerful nutrient that affects learning, memory, attention span and helps to lower anxiety). It also contains B vitamins and calcium, CoQ10 (known to prevent strokes) and protein. One cup gives you 19 grams of protein in this brain stimulator.

Where to buy it: At the grocery store. Canned in olive oil is fine.

How much to eat: Sardines may not seem sexy, but eating just 3 ounces of sardines two or three times a week will give you tremendous dietary value in a tasty, all-natural, low-calorie package.

Quick Facts: There's actually no such fish as a sardine. "Sardine" is a term that refers to a variety of small fish (of various species) that have been processed and canned. The name derives from the Mediterranean island of Sardinia.

Quick Recipe: Sardine Tostada

Quick Recipe: Sardines atop a bed of vegetable greens, black beans, sliced avocado, sun-dried tomato and feta cheese with an olive oil lemon-garlic dressing.

Steak, Lean Top Sirloin

Why: Eating just three ounces of lean top sirloin will give you 25 grams of protein, containing a high amount of the amino acid tyrosine, excellent for brain stimulation. Plus, lean top sirloin beef steak contains niacin (which increases blood circulation in the brain), folic acid, B12, selenium, choline, calcium, iron, magnesium and zinc. There aren't too many Superfoods that are as easy to prepare, as compact (only 3 ounces) and filled with the brain nutrients for sustained concentration throughout the day.

Where to buy it: At your favorite supermarket and if you can buy organic, grass-fed beef you'll get even higher nutrient values.

How much to eat: Three ounces of lean beef, two to three times a week.

Quick Tip: While enjoying your steak, add a side of wild rice mixed with brown rice, a green leafy salad with olive oil balsamic vinegar dressing and an eight ounce glass of red wine for some antioxidant protection. This meal combo will slow digestion and keep a steady flow of energy going to the brain.

Strawberries

Why: Researchers have found that strawberries protect the brain from oxidative stress, reduce the effects of the age-related decline in brain function and significantly improve learning capacity and motor skills. Strawberries are an excellent source of antioxidants, as well as vitamins C and E. This Superfood also qualifies as a good source of dietary fiber, and is high in potassium, magnesium, calcium and folic acid-good for vascular health, concentration and much-needed brain oxygen.

Where to buy it: At the grocery store in either the fresh produce section or frozen section-either way is great. Buy frozen fruits that are flash frozen without any water or sugar syrups added.

How much to take: A ½ cup counts as one of the daily recommended 8 to 10 servings of fruits or vegetables.

Quick Tip: A member of the rose family, there are more than 600 varieties of strawberries that differ in flavor, size and texture and they're the only fruit with seeds on the outside, averaging 200 per strawberry.

Walnuts

Why: Look at this gem closely; it even looks like a brain! Walnuts are rich in protein, providing nine grams in a ¼ cup. They contain a full complement of vitamins, including B1, B2, B3, B5, B6 and folic acid-especially important for energy production in the brain. Walnuts are a rich source of minerals including iron, magnesium, potassium and zinc—all important nutrients for memory. They also contain high amounts of antioxidants, ellagic acid, selenium, CoQ10 and vitamin E—all helping to protect the brain from burn-out. High in polyunsaturates, walnut oil is rich in gamma-tocopherol, a form of vitamin E considered nutritionally superior. (Gamma-tocopherol also protects the oil from becoming rancid too quickly.)

Where to buy it: At the grocery store, either whole, shelled or even as oil.

How much to eat: Three tablespoons of walnut oil will provide our daily requirement of omega-3 fatty acids, or eat ¼ cup of shelled walnuts daily.

Quick recipe: Combine spinach leaves with walnuts, parmesan cheese, raisins, hard boiled egg and extra virgin olive oil for the perfect brain enhancer. A side of brown rice ensures you have enough brain power for the afternoon or evening. Later, impress your partner by blasting through all the answers on Jeopardy.

Wheat Germ

Why: The "germ" is the vitamin and mineral-rich embryo of the wheat kernel that is removed during the refining of whole wheat grains to white flour. Packed with important B vitamins such as folate, thiamin and vitamin B6, and the minerals calcium, iron, potassium, selenium, zinc, magnesium and manganese, wheat germ is packed with brain-stimulating nutrients. You don't need to eat a lot of wheat germ daily- a ½ cup offers 13 grams of tyrosine-rich protein for quick thinking and sustained vascular protection.

Where to buy it: Grocery stores or health food stores carry it in powder or oil form. Either form of wheat germ does the trick–it's your personal preference.

How much to eat: Two to three tablespoons at least four to five days a week.

 Quick Tip: With its nutty flavor, wheat germ is great on top of hot cereals or added to a protein shake. Two to three tablespoons contain about 6 to 9 grams of protein, 2 to 3 grams of unsaturated fat and 2 to 3 grams of fiber.

Yogurt

Why: Yogurt is high in calcium (an important nutrient for mental concentration) and is high in protein (providing fuel for our neurotransmitters). Yogurt also contains magnesium, potassium, zinc and vitamins B12 and folic acid. These nutrients help provide oxygen to the brain, cellular energy and improved concentration.

Where to buy it: There are many yogurts on the market; my favorite is *Stonyfield* because it's organic, has live probiotics and comes in either soy or milk cultures.

How much to eat: Eat 4 to 6 ounces daily.

Quick Tip: Yogurt is relatively high in the amino acid tyrosine (stimulating the brain) and low in the amino acid tryptophan (calming the brain). Add yogurt to other brain foods, such as walnuts and wheat germ, and you have three synergistic foods that form the basics for a cerebral day!

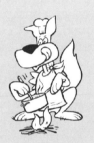

Quick Recipe

- ⅓ cup frozen shelled edamame soy beans or 1 scoop soy isolate protein powder
- ½ cup plain nonfat yogurt
- 1 serving of a high quality superfood drink
- ⅓ cup blueberries or strawberries or blackberries (can be frozen but avoid fruits frozen in syrup)
- 2 Tbls lecithin granules
- 2 Tbls walnut oil
- 2 Tbls peanut butter or almond butter
- 1 tsp cinnamon powder
- 3 Tbls freshly ground flax seed and/or 3 Tbls of oat or wheat bran

Combine all the ingredients in a blender until smooth. Serve immediately after blending while the mixture still has a bubbly, milkshake-like consistency.

Water

Why: Every function inside the body is regulated by and depends on water. Water is essential to carry vital elements, oxygen, hormones and chemical messengers to all parts of the body. In fact, scientists have found that the brain's gray matter is 80% water, and the white matter is 70% water. Without sufficient water to hydrate all parts of your body equally, some of the remote parts of the body will not receive vital water supplies.

> *Quick Facts:* Dr. F. Batmanghelidj's research has found that without sufficient water to constantly hydrate all parts of the body, your drought-management system kicks into action. The histamine-directed chemical messenger systems are activated to arrange a new, lower quota of water for the drought-stricken areas. When histamine and its subordinate "drought managers" come across pain-sensing nerves, they cause pain (i.e. back and joint pain). If dehydration persists, and is not corrected, it becomes symptom-producing and, in time, develops into a disease condition.

Where to buy it: This incredible liquid is found right in your own house (or you can have it delivered).

How much to drink: Here's an easy way to figure out how much water you should drink each day: Drink at least ½ your body weight in ounces; i.e. 150 pounds divided in half = 75 pounds. Next, convert that to ounces = 75 ounces/day. A medium-sized bottle of water is approximately 25 ounces. Try to drink **three** of those each day. It doesn't hurt to drink more water, so if you want more, drink more!

> *Quick Facts:* A mere 2% drop in body water can trigger fuzzy, short-term memory, trouble with basic math and difficulty focusing on the computer screen or on a printed page.

Herbs for Brain Function

Gingko Biloba

Why: More evidence exists for the beneficial effect of ginkgo on mental function than for any other herb. There are more than 300 studies (double-blind, placebo-controlled) on humans that study the effects of ginkgo on mental health. Studies indicate that gingko biloba keeps blood vessels and capillaries flexible, aiding in the circulation of blood, which means that the brain gets a better supply of oxygen, glucose (blood sugar), and nutrients. It also normalizes, or boosts, the levels of certain neurotransmitters.

Where to buy it: At any health food store. Most ginkgo biloba supplements are in an extract form and this is what you want to purchase. It ensures you're getting the maximum benefits for your brain.

How much to take: To enhance brain power, take 60–120 mg daily. Ideally, mix gingko biloba with other brain foods, but it's also fine to take alone on an empty stomach.

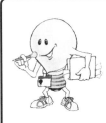

Quick Tip 1: Gingko biloba is a powerful antioxidant, protecting our cells from damage. Brain cells that are protected result in stronger and healthier brain cell membranes.

Quick Tip 2: Gingko is a blood thinner. If you are taking blood thinning medicines, be sure to check with your physician before taking gingko biloba.

Rosemary

Why: The herb rosemary has long been regarded as an herb for remembrance. It increases blood flow to the head and brain, improving concentration, and it's thought to prevent the breakdown of neural transmitters in the brain. It's also a great antioxidant-some studies have found that rosemary has ten times the antioxidant potency of vitamin E.

Where to buy it: In the fresh produce section (in the herb area), at a health food store as a tea or order dried rosemary from www.mountainrose.com.

How much to eat: A tea made from this herb, taken once or twice a day, is a refreshing drink and an effective natural remedy for enhancing mental agility. When using fresh rosemary, break off two, 3-inch stems. Pour one cup boiling water over stems and let stand for 10 minutes. For the dried herb, use 1 teaspoon to 1 cup boiling water and let stand for 10 minutes.

Quick Tip: Rosemary is easy to grow. During the holiday season you can find rosemary plants at local hardware stores–trimmed to look like a Christmas tree. The next time you see one, buy it, plant it and you'll have rosemary for years to come.

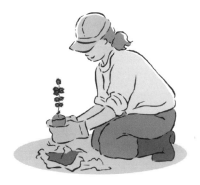

Nutrients For Brain Function

Antioxidants

Antioxidants battle the damage caused by free radicals that may lead to cloudy thought and confusion.

Vitamin C

Vitamin C intake benefits mood, cognitive function and anxiety. Preliminary evidence even suggests that supplements of vitamin C are a valuable adjunctive therapy for schizophrenia.

Quick Fact: A 1993 report from the Department of Psychiatry at Albert Einstein College of Medicine, Bronx, NY found that a 37-year-old chronic schizophrenic patient derived substantial benefits from the addition of ascorbic acid (vitamin C) to his other treatments.

CO Q 10

Coenzyme Q10 (when used in conjunction with vitamin E) improves learning ability.

Selenium

A powerful antioxidant, selenium protects the brain from heavy metals such as lead (used in pipes) and mercury (part of the amalgam used in dental fillings). Even small amounts of heavy metals can accumulate in the tissues and interfere with brain chemistry.

B Vitamins

Probably the most important for optimal brain health, B vitamins are water-soluble which means they're not stored in the body for long; consequently, you need to replenish supplies frequently. B vitamins are vital for brain function, a healthy nervous system and energy metabolism. They are important in the production of the brain neurotransmitters (messengers) dopamine, adrenaline, noradrenaline and serotonin. Poor concentration and memory, lack of energy, insomnia and irritability are signs of a possible deficiency. Niacin is one of the nutrient molecules that is necessary for the proper function of the enzyme called mono-amine oxidase (MAO).

EFAs

Eating foods high in essential fatty acids (EFAs) and most importantly, high in DHA (the primary structural component of brain tissue) helps the brain cells better communicate with each other.

DHA affects three main areas of brain function: (1) mood and behavior; (2) cognition (learning, memory, etc.); and (3) movement and sensation. Plus, EFAs help prevent blood clotting in the brain.

Quick Facts: New evidence shows that the body cannot make adequate amounts of DHA. However, eating oily fish, like salmon, twice a week will provide a modest intake of DHA. Add a fish oil supplement high in omega-3 fatty acids to ensure a steady and adequate supply. For the vegetarian: DHA derived from marine algae is a good alternative.

Choline

Choline is converted in the body to acetylcholine, regulating memory and mental sharpness. Because of choline's role in the production of acetylcholine (a neurotransmitter responsible for coordination), a deficiency may lead to impaired muscle coordination. Also most people who are affected by cluster headaches exhibit a deficiency in choline levels.

DMAE

DMAE elevates one's mood, counters depression, boosts cognitive functions and even increases intelligence. These benefits stem from this brain nutrient's role in manufacturing the crucial neurotransmitter acetylcholine.

Quick facts: One of the best measures of cognitive function is reaction time. How quickly can you make a decision under pressure or in a crisis?

Folic Acid

Folic acid helps maintain the brain's levels of memory. It has been found that low levels of folic acid may contribute to impaired concentration, abstract reasoning, dementia, depression and insomnia. Also, pregnant woman who are low in folic acid may have an increased risk in giving birth to a child with Downs Syndrome.

Calcium

Not just good for bones, calcium increases your ability to concentrate. Approximately 22% of autism patients are found to be deficient in calcium and many parents report that their autistic children respond favorably to calcium supplementation. Calcium may also prove useful in the prevention/treatment of Alzheimer's disease.

Quick Facts: In the 2000 edition of *Vitamin Research News*, the author speculated that calcium deficiency may be an underlying cause of ADD. Children who are deficient in calcium experience irritability, sleep disturbances, aggressiveness and inattentiveness (all symptoms of ADD). This is not the only answer to solving the ever-growing epidemic of ADD, but adding more calcium to children's diet may help.

Iron

This important mineral transports oxygen through the red blood cells, including those that travel to your brain. Iron-poor blood is linked to a short attention span and mental sluggishness. An iron deficiency starves the brain of oxygen and interferes with cognition–long before clinical anemia develops. Iron supplements, in addition to alleviating many of the physical complications of iron deficiency, may even improve some basic cognitive functions such as memory and ability to learn.

Magnesium

Low levels of magnesium in the diet can lead to decreased attention span, poor concentration ability, mental confusion and loss of coordination. In research conducted at the Eotvos University, Hungary in 2000, magnesium levels were found to be significantly decreased in brain regions of Alzheimer's patients. And magnesium may also be beneficial to ADD children. A study conducted showed there was a significant decrease in hyperactive behavior when magnesium levels were raised.

Potassium

Potassium facilitates the transport of oxygen to the brain.

Zinc

Crucial for memory and brain function, zinc is important in the synthesis of the brain-calming chemical serotonin.

Boron

Boron has been found to aid memory and improve attention and mental alertness and is essential for energy metabolism.

Proteins

Protein's amino acids provide fuel for our neurotransmitters. Neurotransmitters carry signals from one brain cell to another. These cells, called neurons, are organized to control specialized activities like thinking and feeling.

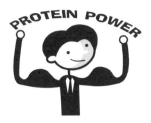

Proteins are sometimes described as long necklaces with differently shaped beads. Each bead is a small molecule called an amino acid. The amino acids maintain muscles, bones, blood and body organs. Amino acids join together to make thousands of different proteins, but 22 of them are very important to human health. Of those 22 amino acids, your body can make 13 of them without you ever even thinking about it. Your body can't make the other nine amino acids, so you must get them by eating protein-rich foods. They're called **essential amino acids** because it's **essential** that you get them from the foods you eat.

Protein's amino acids provide fuel for our neurotransmitters. Neurotransmitters carry signals from one brain cell to another. These cells, called neurons, are organized to control specialized activities like thinking and feeling. Some neurotransmitters calm you down, while others keep you on the ball. The two important amino acids, **tryptophan** and **tyrosine**, are vital in the production of neurotransmitters. Tryptophan must come from the foods you eat. Your body can make tyrosine if you don't consume enough in your diet. Consuming proteins that contain higher tyrosine amino acids can keep you more alert, whereas eating proteins that contain high tryptophan amino acids (combined with high carbohydrate foods) will help you relax.

The Perfect Combination of Carbs & Protein for Brain Power

Three factors influence whether the brain perks up or slows down following a meal: (1) the ratio of carbohydrates to proteins consumed; (2) whether the proteins contain more tyrosine or more tryptophan; and (3) the amount of calories in the meal.

To stimulate your brain, combine a high tyrosine-containing protein (sardines, walnuts, beef steak, pork chops) with a complex carbohydrate (brown rice, quinoa, oatmeal), and make it low calorie. Combining complex carbohydrates that slow down the release of insulin, with proteins that are high in tyrosine, will stimulate the brain and help it perform on a more sustained level. A low-calorie, high-protein meal that contains complex carbohydrates keeps you more alert and would be perfect for breakfast and lunch.

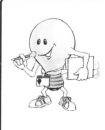

Quick Tip 1: Playing men against the women in a game of Cranium™ tonight? You may want to stimulate your brain first! Eat a simple snack like peanut butter with sliced apples and a handful of walnuts to get the upper edge. Eating less gives you more brain power. If your hunger is greater than apples and peanut butter can satisfy, try making a tuna salad sandwich on high grain wheat bread, add some romaine lettuce, sliced tomato and egg mayonnaise. But eat only one sandwich if you want to be on top of your game!

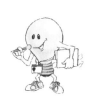

Quick Tip 2: The balance between calories, carbohydrates and protein in a meal affects different people in different ways. This is not an exact science. You need to figure out which combinations work the best for you, giving you energy and alertness when you need it. Some people need more calories to function because they have higher metabolisms, while others need less. Experiment and adjust your calories accordingly.

Use Your Noodle to Choose Carbohydrates

The brain is the ultimate sugar junkie; it loves and craves carbohydrates, utilizing a whopping 20 percent of the body's carbohydrate supply. But it is selective about the type of sugars it craves and how it processes them, preferring a nice, steady supply. When levels of sugar in the blood rise and fall, the brain doesn't get its steady fuel supply, and behavior and learning can become more erratic. Creating a steady supply depends on the kinds of food you eat. The results can be stimulating (enhancing your imagination or memories), or calming and sedating.

What's a Complex Carb? A+

Complex carbs are referred to as polysaccharides (long chains of sugar molecules bonded together) and are found in foods like fruits, vegetables, legumes (peas and beans), and grains (quinoa, buckwheat and rice). Some are also referred to as dietary starches. These are mostly from the grain family and include cereals, breads, pasta, oats, wheat, rice and corn, but are also found in some vegetables like potatoes and legumes.

What's a Simple Carb? C-

Simple carbs are just that-the simplest form of carbs. These are found as either single sugar molecules referred to as monosaccharides, (glucose, fructose or galactose) or naturally occurring sugars found in most fruits, honey and milk. Simple carbs are also double sugar molecules, referred to as disaccharides (sucrose, maltose and lactose). The majority of disaccharides come from man-made, processed sugars. Avoid these whenever you can.

> *Quick Facts: Brain Drainers:* Consuming alcohol, artificial sweeteners, colas, corn syrup, high sugar drinks, hydrogenated fats, junk food, sugars, white bread, nicotine and even overeating can drain your body of valuable nutrients needed for powering your brain!

The Glycemic Index

The body breaks down most carbohydrates from the foods we eat and converts them to a type of sugar called glucose. Glucose is the main source of fuel for our cells. After eating, the time it takes for the body to convert carbohydrates and release glucose into the bloodstream varies depending on the type of carbohydrate and the food. Some carbohydrate-containing foods cause the blood glucose level to rise rapidly. Others have a more gradual effect. Foods with higher index values raise blood sugar more rapidly than foods with lower glycemic index values. The glycemic index (GI) measures how fast and how much a food raises blood glucose levels.

Foods with a high GI stimulate the pancreas to secrete a lot of insulin, which causes the sugar to quickly empty from the blood into the cells; this fast emptying of sugar produces the ups and downs of blood sugar and the roller coaster behavior that goes with them. Foods with a low GI do not push the pancreas to secrete an overload of insulin, so the blood sugar tends to be steadier, creating a sustained energy level.

Quick Tip: Low glycemic index fruits are grapefruit, apples, pears, cherries and peaches. Barley, all bran, brown rice, wild rice or milk and yogurt are also low glycemic foods. **Legumes (beans) such as soybeans, lentils, kidney beans, black beans and chick peas have the lowest glycemic index of any food.**

P.S. Don't Forget to Exercise Your Mind... Research shows exercising the brain is equally as important as exercising the body. Stimulation from puzzles, learning a new language, playing an instrument, or even just having stimulating conversations can expand the brain to process information more quickly.

Quick Tip:
Try www.brainbashers.com or www.brainbusters.com for Web sites full of fun, cerebral games.

...And Exercise Your Body Too

There is clear evidence that an aerobic exercise program, even a fairly gentle one, may boost performance in key areas of the brain helping with decision-making and focus. Physical activity helps improve the blood flow to the brain and stimulates the release of chemicals that influence brain cell growth and activity.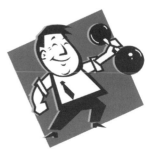

- ✓ Jumping rope might be the best exercise for preparing the brain to learn because it uses different areas of the brain, performing several tasks simultaneously.
- ✓ Getting up from your desk and going for a brisk walk may help keep your mind agile later in life.
- ✓ Aerobics, doing a puzzle or just learning something new can increase your mental capacity by three to five years!
- ✓ Deep-breathing, used in exercises like Yoga, gets much-needed oxygen to the brain.

Quick Facts:
A recent study showed that when people followed a diet:
- low on meat
- low on dairy products
- heavy on fish
- heavy on fruits
- heavy on vegetables
- heavy on monounsaturated fats found in cod liver oil, olive oil and avocados

had a **40% lower risk** of developing Alzheimer's disease than those who ate a conventional American diet.

Quick Facts: Brain research is beginning to produce concrete evidence for something that Buddhist practitioners of meditation have maintained for centuries: Mental discipline and meditative practice can change the workings of the brain and allow people to achieve different levels of awareness.

Chapter 2

. . . .

Superfoods for Moods and Stress

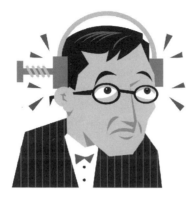

Your life is filled with deadlines, over-scheduling and much multi-tasking. The demands you place on your body and mind can easily lead to a quick-fix mentality. Coffee, sugar and that menacing combination of the triple-shot, caramel macchiato are the quick fixes that provide the quick highs-and even quicker lows. That satisfied feeling rapidly plummets, resulting in a frenetic search for the next drive-thru espresso stand. It's a vicious cycle! But relax, because a few key foods and supplements will wipe away fatigue and reduce stress without wiping you out (or your wallet).

A few simple adjustments to your diet may do wonders for your emotional well being. What and when we eat has an overwhelming influence on brain chemistry and a direct connection on how we think and act. How we respond to stress depends as much on diet as it does on learned coping skills. Combining the right Superfoods throughout the day is one great start, plus: (1) Eat a diet high in complex carbohydrates with a low glycemic index (legumes and unrefined grains have a balancing effect as they cause fewer blood sugar disturbances); (2) Consume protein three times a day to help with depression and anxiety–proteins will help to keep blood sugar levels consistent; (3) Add proteins with high tryptophan amino acids such as pumpkin and sunflower seeds and parmesan cheese, that aid in the creation of serotonin and endorphins (mood regulating neurotransmitters); and (4) Eat foods high in B vitamins. Eating junk food for a few days, while tense and stressed, can lead to a vitamin B deficiency–quickly compounding the problem.

Don't Worry, Be Happy

- ✓ By cutting your sleep short, you **limit the growth of new brain cells**.
- ✓ Most adults need eight to nine hours of sleep per night to maintain proper health.
- ✓ Chronic stress robs you of brain power. It literally *shrinks and destroys* the brain regions that are crucial for memory.
- ✓ When romantic relationships end, the results can be devastating. It's found to be similar to the same brain changes as a person who is going through Post-Traumatic Stress Disorder (PTSD), affecting both motivation and attention.
- ✓ 75% of the U.S. population experiences at least some signs of stress in their lives every two weeks.
- ✓ Stress contributes to heart disease, high blood pressure, strokes and other illnesses.
- ✓ Stress affects our immune system, leaving us less protected from many serious diseases.
- ✓ Tranquilizers, antidepressants and anti-anxiety medications account for ¼ of all prescriptions written in the U.S. each year.

Superfoods for Mood Enhancing and Stress Reducing

Beets

Why: A number of compounds in foods have been shown to raise serotonin levels and induce a subsequent calming effect in patients suffering from depression. Betaine, found in beets, is also known as trimethylglycine (TMG). Treatment with betaine (TMG) raises levels of a compound called s-adenosylmethionine (SAMe), which in turn influences serotonin metabolism. Betaine is a mood modifier. In the diet, betaine-rich foods are pharmacologically active, and can have a positive effect on mood by relaxing the mind. Beetroot, because it contains betaine, is therefore a minor "mood food."

Where to buy it: At the grocery store in the fresh produce section or canned section. Finding fresh beetroot is always the first choice, but consuming canned beets is better than not eating them at all!

How much to eat: A ½ cup is only 37 calories. Make this one of your daily 8 to 10 servings of vegetables and fruits a day, three to four times a week.

Quick Tip: Beetroot has unique chemicals (e.g. betalains and betaine) and high levels of important micronutrients. The betalains act as antioxidants. Betaine is a dietary antioxidant with a particularly high bioavailability, with very little being excreted under normal conditions. Just a little beetroot is beneficial. Plus, it has other antioxidant nutrients including vitamin C and beta-carotene, which help fight infection and help detoxify a range of carcinogenic chemicals.

Black Beans

Why: Black beans are high in fiber, complex carbs and protein. This all-in-one combination prevents blood sugar levels from rising too rapidly, supplies protein that stops cravings for sugar and junk food and contributes to stabilizing stress. Black beans are also filled with nutrients that directly contribute to brain health, giving you the ability to cope with a high stress lifestyle.

Where to buy it: In the dried beans section of your grocery store. If you don't have the time to prepare dried black beans, canned are an option.

How much to eat: One cup of black beans will provide you with 15.2 grams of protein (the average body needs around 70 grams of protein daily). Substituting black beans for higher fat foods (such as red meat) for one meal daily would be ideal.

Speedy preparation: Dried black beans cook much more quickly if soaked in water over night. After soaking, rinse beans, add water (one cup beans to four cups water) bring water to a boil and add beans; they'll be ready in 30 minutes. To help reduce the foaming while beans cook, add one tablespoon of oil. Here's a trick to help reduce the feeling of gas that is sometimes produced from eating beans: add a couple bay leaves to the pot while cooking.

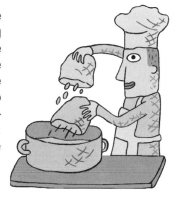

Quick Recipe
Spice Up Your Mood Black Bean Salad

Mix in a bowl:
- 1 cup cooked black beans
- ½ cup diced tomatoes
- ⅓ cup shredded Swiss or gruyere cheese
- ¼ cup diced red bell peppers
- ¼ cup chopped green onions
- ¼ cup chopped fresh cilantro
- 1 Tbls olive oil
- 1 Tbls lime juice
- ½ tsp ground cumin
- 3 cups shopped fresh spinach
- Salt and pepper to taste

The darker the bean's coat, the higher level of antioxidants.

Chocolate

Why: Researchers have found that eating dark chocolate (the number one food craved by American women) causes the brain to release endorphins–chemicals that make us feel good. It is believed there are a few combined substances that actually create this psychochemical effect. They produce the endorphins, believed to contribute to the renowned "inner glow" experienced by dedicated chocolate lovers. Chocolate also contains chemical compounds, like flavonoids, also found in wine, that have antioxidant properties and reduce serum cholesterol.

Quick Facts: The human body produces at least 20 different endorphins. Endorphins are believed to produce four key effects on the body/mind: (1) enhance the immune system, (2) relieve pain, (3) reduce stress and (4) postpone the aging process. Scientists also have found that beta-endorphins can activate human NK (Natural Killer) cells and boost the immune system. Researchers continue to investigate endorphins' many benefits and uses.

Where to buy it: Who doesn't know where to find chocolate?! You can find it almost anywhere: grocery stores, department stores, specialty chocolate shops, gas stations and convenient stores.

How much to eat: The best chemical-producing chocolate is dark chocolate. This delicacy is high in fat, so eating as little as one ounce is enough to be beneficial.

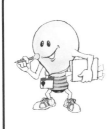 *Quick Tip:* Naturally produced by the body, endorphins are possibly the best way to achieve a natural high. Chemically speaking, endorphins are polypeptides, which bind to the neuro-receptors in the brain to give relief from pain. First discovered in 1975, endorphins ("endogenous morphine") are one of several morphine-like substances (opioids) discovered within our brains. Opioids are considered stress hormones and are manufactured by the body to reduce stress and relieve pain. Usually produced during periods of extreme stress, endorphins naturally block pain signals.

Gruyere Cheese (groo•YEHR)

Why: Gruyere is high in the amino acid tryptophan that produces serotonin, an important neurotransmitter in the brain that keeps us focused and calm. It also is an excellent source of other essentials—a ½ cup will provide you with calcium (667 mg) and magnesium (24 mg), known nutrients to help prevent anxiety. Plus, it's the perfect protein source, contains many of the B vitamins and is high in zinc (an important mineral often found low in people with depression).

Where to buy it: At the grocery store in the dairy aisle or specialty cheese section.

How much to eat: Eat a ¼ cup, once or twice daily.

 Quick Tip 1: Named for the Swiss village that produces it, gruyere is the basic ingredient in fondue, but can also be substituted for Swiss cheese in your favorite dish. Because it melts easily, it works in grilled sandwiches, soufflés or as a topping on soups. It's made from cow's milk and noted for its smooth, nutty flavor. Look for its distinctive small holes, similar to Swiss cheese.

 Quick Tip 2: Snack on a small plate of sliced gruyere cheese, fresh or dried figs, pumpkin seeds and a few whole wheat baked crackers.

Mustard Greens

Why: Mustard greens may not be your first choice, but they are extremely nutritious, offering a high amount of B vitamins needed to promote a steady supply of nutrients for healthy neurotransmitter production (controlling stress levels). Plus, they are high in the minerals manganese, copper, magnesium, calcium, potassium and phosphorous—all necessary for relaxed muscles, anti-depression and memory enhancement. In addition to all the nutrients listed, mustard greens are extremely high in vitamin A, the *antioxidants* lutein and zeaxanthin and vitamin C.

Where to buy it: In the fresh produce section of the grocery store. Mustard greens have either a crumpled or flat texture and may have either toothed, scalloped, frilled or lacey edges. Look for mustard greens that are free of brown spots, yellowing and blemishes.

How much to eat: A ½ cup equals one of the daily recommended 8 to 10 servings of vegetables and fruits.

Speedy preparation: Rinse the greens in water, fold them in half and remove the stem. Greens can be added to salad or chopped and added to soup, pasta or any dish in need of a little spice. Remember, it's the combinations of Superfoods that contribute to stabilizing moods and stress. Add some gruyere cheese, pumpkin seeds, black beans and a little extra virgin olive oil with your fresh mustard greens for a great lunch or afternoon snack

Nutritional Yeast

Why: Eating nutritional yeast is an easy way to get all of the B vitamins needed to keep stress levels under control and it provides the nutrients to make SAMe (necessary for serotonin, melatonin, and dopamine production). In addition, nutritional yeast is high in protein, niacin and B6 (which lessens irritability and keeps the mind focused). Nutritional yeast contains no dairy products, sugar or preservatives.

Where to buy it: At any health food store; ask for a recommendation for the best-tasting nutritional yeast they carry, like *RedStar*. Don't confuse nutritional yeast with brewer's yeast or yeast for baking.

How much to eat: Eat 2 tablespoons per day.

Speedy preparation: It doesn't get any easier than this. Nutritional yeast can simply be added to any beverage. Add, stir and drink up!

 Quick Tip 1: For a great tasting, nutritious snack: dust nutritional yeast liberally over hot popcorn. Sprinkle it over spaghetti, pizza or other dishes as a healthy replacement for grated cheese. You can also use it as a seasoning for salads, sauces, gravies, soups, casseroles, burgers and spreads.

Quick Tip 2: Nutritional yeast is dried at high temperature which inactivates the yeast content. In other words, you can't use this to raise bread. It's cultivated specifically for use as a supplement.

Quinoa (Keen•wah)

Why: Quinoa, a grain, supplies a complete protein (providing all nine essential amino acids), and is a great source of complex carbs. The combo keeps blood sugar levels balanced, guarding against those highs and lows throughout the day. A favorite, this Superfood is delicious when eaten cold or hot and provides the brain with nutrients to maintain stability when feeling tense. Its high mineral concentrations of magnesium, manganese, copper, calcium and iron help maintain focus and relaxation.

Where to buy it: If you can't find it in your local supermarket, look for it at natural foods stores. Quinoa is sometimes found in bins or prepackaged in the dried bean section.

How much to take: Eating one cup will help satisfy those carbohydrate cravings plus give you protein. This is a great source of protein among other nutrients, alternating with black beans, soy beans and other high protein non meat foods will give you the essential amino acids necessary to stabilize moods and stress levels.

Quick Tip 1: Cook quinoa like rice: 1 cup quinoa to 2 cups water. Using a rice cooker makes this an easy dish to prepare. Add ¼ teaspoon of your favorite spices to the water while cooking. My favorites are cumin, curry, grated orange peel, cloves, cinnamon or nutmeg. Quinoa has a fluffy, creamy, slightly crunchy texture and a somewhat nutty flavor.

Quick Tip 2: Quinoa is a great substitute for refined pastas (which offer little nutritional value). Ground quinoa flour can be added to cookie or muffin recipes instead of refined flour.

Quick Tip 3: If you are prone to migraines, try adding quinoa to your diet. Quinoa is a good source of magnesium, a mineral that helps relax blood vessels, preventing the constriction and rebound dilation characteristic of migraines. Quinoa is also a good source of riboflavin (also called vitamin B2), shown to reduce the frequency of attacks in migraine sufferers.

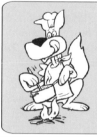

Quick Recipe

Combine cooked quinoa with black beans, pumpkin seeds, diced dried fruits, scallions and coriander. Season with salt, pepper or curry spices to taste and enjoy this south-of-the-border-inspired salad.

Pumpkin Seeds

Why: Also known as pepitas, pumpkin seeds are one of the richest source of minerals. They are high in tryptophan protein (for serotonin production) and contain good monounsaturated fat (for brain health) creating the perfect relaxing snack food. They're a well balanced nutrient-rich source of the minerals magnesium, manganese, phosphorous, iron and copper and, you guessed it–they contribute to calming nerves while lifting your spirits. Snacking on a handful of roasted pumpkin seeds may be the perfect prescription for calming nerves.

Where to buy them: Grocery store or specialty markets–either salted, unsalted raw or roasted. If you have a Trader Joe's Market near you, they offer a good selection of packaged pepitas (pumpkin seeds) to choose from.

How much to eat: ¼ cup daily is a great addition to other healthy nuts and seeds.

Quick Tip: Pumpkin seeds (pepitas) are flat, green seeds, usually shelled. If you purchase raw, you can roast them easily by spreading them on a cookie sheet and putting them under the broiler in your oven. Don't cook them too close to the heat; they'll start popping like popcorn. It only takes about five minutes to brown them; so watch them closely. They taste so good warm that it will be hard not to eat the whole pan in a single sitting! By adding a few dried cranberries or raisins to your mix, you quicken the insulin response, helping tryptophan get to your brain quicker.

Tuna

Why: Tuna fish is truly a nutrient-dense food, high in protein and the B vitamins niacin, B1 and B6–necessary nutrients to make SAMe (a needed component for serotonin and melatonin production). Plus, tuna is rich in the minerals magnesium and potassium, known to help prevent muscle tightness usually associated with stress. Tuna is also a great source of omega-3s that contribute to high performance brain function.

Where to buy it: At any grocery store, both canned and fresh tuna are available throughout the year. Water packed light canned tuna is the best choice.

How much to eat: Eat one 3 to 6 ounce portion of fish three to four times per week.

 Quick Tip 1: Eating fish, like tuna, as little as one to three times per month has been found to protect against ischemic stroke, a stroke caused by lack of blood supply to the brain.

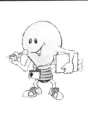 ***Quick Tip 2:*** A study published in the January 2004 issue of the *European Journal of Clinical Nutrition* found a statistically significant relationship between consuming fish rich in omega-3 fats and lower hostility scores in 3,581 young urban adults. Those with the highest intake of omega-3 fats had only a 10% likelihood of having the highest hostility scores. A second reason this finding is important: hostility has been shown to predict the development of heart disease.

Winter Squash

Why: There aren't many vegetables that can claim the nutrient value of winter squash; it is high in B vitamins (quickly lost when under stress), omega-3s and potassium. These nutrients, in combination, are thought to help relieve anxiety. It has also been found that low levels of potassium can create nervousness. Most winter squash also have the *antioxidant* protection of vitamin A, C and E.

Where to buy it: At the grocery store in the fresh produce section. If you can't find fresh, frozen winter squash found in the freezer section is a good alternative.

How much to take? A ½ cup counts as one of the daily recommended 8 to 10 servings of vegetables and fruits.

 Quick Tip: Varieties of winter squash are:
- Butternut squash (with a cream-colored skin, deep orange-colored flesh and a sweet flavor)
- Acorn squash (with a unique sweet, nutty and peppery flavor; its skin is green with speckled orange patches and light yellow-orange flesh)
- Hubbard squash (not as sweet, larger than the others with a dark green skin or sometimes orange in color)
- Turban squash (tastes similar to hazelnuts with a green speckled or striped skin)

Quick Tip: The best way to prepare winter squash is to bake it. Cut in quarters, remove the seeds and bake approximately 30 minutes. If desired, brush it gently with butter or oil. Adding crushed pistachio nuts on top not only makes it taste great, it gives you a good portion of protein.

Water, Water, Water!

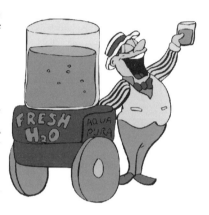

Why: Studies link depression to dehydration because over 80% of brain tissue consists of water. Dehydration causes decreased energy generation in the brain, so a lack of water can be the culprit in many disorders, and it is the number one trigger for daytime fatigue. A mere 2% drop in water can trigger fuzzy, short-term memory, trouble with basic math and difficulty focusing on the computer screen or on a printed page.

Where to buy it: You can find this incredible liquid right in your own house!

How much to drink: Here's an easy way to figure out how much water you should drink each day: Drink at least ½ your body weight in ounces, i.e., 150 pounds divided in half = 75 pounds; next, convert that to ounces = 75 ounce/day. A medium sized bottle of water is approximately 25 ounces. Try to drink three of those each day. Remember: it's perfectly safe to drink more!

 Quick Tip 1: There are several types of anxiety disorders, the most common being General Anxiety Disorder (GAD). When the body is dehydrated it can actually induce anxiety and nervousness. Beverages with caffeine also increase anxiety. Replacing soda, tea and coffee with water is a good start in reducing anxiety.

 Quick Tip 2: Aside from drinking water, hydrotherapy is a calming remedy for stress and anxiety. Taking a warm bath with an herbal supplement can do wonders for the body and soul. It sounds like a cliché, but the hot water will literally ease muscle tension. The soothing herbs and quiet time also allows the mind to escape. You can literally wash those cares away!

A Little Herb Might do Ya ...

Eleuthero (E•leu•ther•o), *Siberian ginseng*

Why: This plant is used as an invigorating tonic to combat stress and fatigue and lower blood sugar levels. Eleuthero is considered an adaptogen, which means that it helps return the body to a normal balance. As an example, an adaptogen might lower blood pressure in someone who has high blood pressure, but raise it in another person who has low blood pressure. Eleuthero purportedly enhances physical endurance and mental concentration.

Where to buy it: Vitamin stores, health food stores and sometimes at your local drug store.

How much to take: It comes in capsule form. Follow the recommended dose on the package.

Hops *Humulus lupulus L.* or *Cannabaceae*

Why: You've probably heard of hops. The bud is used in making beer and acts as a great sedative and relaxant. If you make a hops tea, beware the herb is a little bitter by itself. Adding cinnamon, nutmeg, stevia and a little ginger will improve the taste. If you are of age to drink alcohol, drinking a bottle of beer that is high in hops will actually help you relax.

Where to buy it: Vitamin stores or health food stores.

How much to take: Drink as a tea, two cups a day. Add 1 cup of boiling water over 1 to 2 teaspoons of dried hops flower and steep for 10 minutes.

Passion Flower *Passiflora incarnata*

Why: This is a favorite herb for relaxing. It has an amazing ability to stop the brain from going and going and going, toiling over and over the same thought again and again. It's much more effective than counting sheep! It has a mild flavor and is often combined with chamomile tea and lemon balm to soften its effect.

Where to buy it: Vitamin stores or health food stores.

How much to take: Passion flower is available as a tea or as a tincture. Pour 1 cup of boiling water over 1 to 2 teaspoons of dried passion flower and steep for 10 minutes. Drink up to two cups per day for four to six weeks. Or as a tincture, 10 to 60 drops, three times a day.

Quick Tip: One recent study of 36 men and women with Generalized Anxiety Disorder found that when taken for one month, passion flower was as effective as a leading anti-anxiety medication. A second study, including 91 people with anxiety symptoms, revealed that an herbal European product containing passion flower and other herbal sedatives significantly reduced symptoms. To be safe we can always say it may be advisable to check with your doctor if you are under treatment for depression.

Saint John's Wort *Hypericum perforatum*

Why: Used to treat a range of illnesses, including various nervous conditions and depression, St. John's wort is one of the most commonly purchased herbal products in the United States. Because St. John's wort interacts with a wide variety of medications, it is important to take it only under the guidance of a healthcare provider who is knowledgeable about herbal medicines.

Where to buy it: Vitamin stores, health food stores or your favorite drug store.

How much to take: St. John's wort can be purchased in either capsules or tablet form. The usual dose for mild depression and mood disorders is 300 to 500 mg three times per day, with meals. If you prefer a liquid extract, the recommended dose is 40 to 60 drops, two times per day. It is also available as a tea: pour 1 cup of boiling water over 1 to 2 teaspoons of dried St. John's wort and steep for 10 minutes. Drink up to 2 cups per day for four to six weeks.

Valerian Root (va·le·ri·an)

Why: I call this herb my "heavy hitter." It's used to ease insomnia, stress-related anxiety and nervous restlessness. Valerian is a popular treatment alternative to sleeping medications because it's considered to be both safe and gentle. In studies of animals and people, valerian has demonstrated mild sedative and tranquilizing activity, as well as the ability to relieve anxiety. Generally, valerian reduces the time it takes to fall asleep and improves the quality of sleep itself. Plus, unlike many prescription sleep aids, valerian may have fewer after effects such as morning drowsiness.

Where to buy it: Vitamin stores, health food stores or your favorite drug store.

How much to take: As a tea, pour one cup of boiling water over 1 to 2 teaspoons of dried root and steep for 10 minutes. Drink up to two cups per day. It also comes in capsule or tablet form. Follow the recommended directions on the box or bottle.

Quick Tip: To help bring on sleep, reduce nervousness or anxiety, valerian may be taken an hour or so before bed, or up to three times during the day, with the last dose near bedtime. It may take a few weeks to notice the effects. Once sleep improves, valerian should be continued for two to four weeks. A total of four to six weeks is usually the length of treatment advised by herbalists. After six weeks, a two-week break is recommended to see if natural sleep has improved.

Nutrients for Moods and Stress

Protein

Consuming protein three times a day can help with depression or anxiety and ensure your blood sugar level is balanced. Protein contains the necessary amino acids to create serotonin and endorphins-our mood regulating neurotransmitters.

B Vitamins

B vitamins are necessary for producing SAMe, a component of serotonin, melatonin and dopamine (mood stabilizing neurotransmitters in the brain) production. Often when our bodies are stressed we lose more B vitamins than normal, creating a cycle of not having the nutrients to make chemicals we need to lift our spirits. To compound the problem, many people crave sugary foods and quick-fix junk food to ease the stress. After a few days of this eating behavior, more B vitamins are lost, and the cycle worsens. If you find you're extremely stressed, eating a diet high in B vitamins and protein can help make the shift. If you feel your stress is more severe, consider taking a good time-released B-complex; start with 100mg.

Iron

Iron enhances oxygen distribution throughout the body and is necessary to produce energy. If we lack iron, less hemoglobin is produced meaning less oxygen gets to our brain. And iron has been found to relieve symptoms of tiredness, weakness, irritability and depression.

Quick Tip: **The "Double-Whammy":** Caffeine is often the first thing we reach for when we want a lift in spirits. This habit increases the problem of low iron because caffeine and tannic acid, found in coffee and tea, decrease the absorption of iron! Drinking one or two cups throughout the day is probably safe, but more than that can lead to low iron. Also, iron absorption is decreased in people with low stomach acid, a condition common in the elderly and those who use antacids frequently.

Magnesium

It's been found that increasing magnesium consumption lessens symptoms of depression. When the body gets stressed, some 1,400 chemical changes occur, depleting magnesium. This vital mineral is necessary for energy production, muscle relaxation and calcium absorption. It's also been noted that eating a diet high in fats, phosphorus or calcium decreases absorption.

Zinc and Potassium

Zinc and potassium help relieve low serotonin levels that lead to depression and tension.

Vitamin A and C

Vitamins A and C are two more vitamins depleted during the chemical changes brought on by stress.

Carbohydrates

Being stressed sets off those cravings for carbohydrates, especially the high-sugar ones like cookies, candy bars and ice cream. During times of stress, our body releases hormones that can lower the levels of serotonin in the brain. Carbohydrates make more of these relaxing neurotransmitters in the brain. The key is getting the right kind of carbs (complex carbs).

EFAs

Choosing foods high in EFAs helps balance mood swings and feelings of stress. Adding more foods containing omega-9 (oleic acid) to your daily foods supports the brain's mood-generating activity by affecting the way in which cells are constructed and impacting the flow of serotonin (a mood regulating neurotransmitter) through your brain.

Quick Tip 1: One to two tablespoons of extra virgin or virgin olive oil per day provides sufficient omega-9 (oleic acid) for adults. However, the "time-released" effects of obtaining these nutrients from nuts and other whole foods are thought to be more beneficial.

Quick Tip 2: Eating foods that use MSG (a flavor enhancer/preservative) can actually worsen mood swings. When dining out, ask if they use MSG.

Our Tiny Messengers: Neurotransmiters

The biochemical basis of the food-mood relationship is found in the neurotransmitters, tiny chemical messengers which relay thoughts and actions along the trillions of neural pathways in the brain. Because neurotransmitters are synthesized from the nutrients in our food, what we eat has an overwhelming influence on brain chemistry.

Tryptophan (covered in Chapter One) has two important functions. First, a small amount of the tryptophan we get in our diet (about 3%) is converted into niacin (vitamin B3) by the liver. This conversion can help prevent the symptoms associated with niacin deficiency. Second, tryptophan serves to create serotonin, a neurotransmitter that helps the body regulate appetite, sleep patterns and mood. Because of its ability to raise serotonin levels, tryptophan has been used therapeutically in the treatment of a variety of conditions-most notably insomnia, depression and anxiety.

Vitamin B6 is necessary for the conversion of tryptophan to both niacin and serotonin. In addition, several dietary, lifestyle and health factors reduce the conversion of tryptophan to serotonin, including cigarette smoking, high sugar intake, alcohol abuse, excessive consumption of protein, hypoglycemia and diabetes.

The compound S-Adenosylmethionine (SAMe) helps produce and break down brain chemicals such as serotonin, melatonin and dopamine as well as vitamin B12. SAMe is effective in treating mild to moderate depression and is just as effective as anti-depressant medications (without the side effects). SAMe is not found in food. It is produced by the body from ATP and the amino acid methionine. In order for our body to make SAMe, it needs specific nutrients such as methionine, betaine, folic acid, B12 and B6.

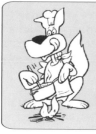

Quick Recipe

Superfood SAMe Sandwich
Layer sliced turkey, watercress, egg yolk mayonnaise and gruyere cheese on whole wheat bread (the bread must be made with wheat germ). Add a couple slices of fresh figs and you have a SAMe nutrient power booster!

Sedate the Brain Meal

Carbohydrates stimulate the release of insulin, moving tryptophan into the brain where it makes more serotonin. Eating a meal that is tryptophan-heavy, with simple sugars that speed-up the release of insulin, creates more production of serotonin, sedating the brain. A high calorie, high carbohydrate, lower protein meal will help you relax and fall asleep; although this maybe not be the smartest choice for weight-watching!

Quick Tip: When it's time to really relax and put aside the things that constitute your stressful life, do it with healthy food. Choose foods that are beautiful to look at and delicious to savor, such as a plate of grapes or strawberries, a wedge of gruyere cheese (or hummus) or some carrot slices to encourage the mind to unwind. Your body will benefit and you enjoy your time with simple, good foods.

Don't Forget To Exercise Your Body
The Great Stress / Mood Stabilizer!

- Exercise is prescribed in clinical settings to help treat nervous tension. Following a session of exercise, clinicians measured a decrease in electrical activity of tensed muscles. People are less jittery and hyperactive following exercise.

- One 30 to 45 minute exercise session generates 90 to 120 minutes of relaxation response. Sometimes called post-exercise euphoria or endorphin response, we now know that many neurotransmitters, not just endorphins, are involved. The important thing, though, is not what they're called, but what they do: They improve your mood and allow you to relax.

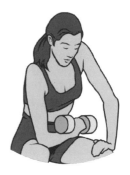

- People who exercise regularly tend to eat more nutritious food. Combined together, good nutrition and exercise is the perfect combination to better manage stress.

Laughter - Fake it
Your Brain Won't Know the Difference!

Studies have shown that laughing lowers blood pressure, reduces stress hormones, increases muscle flexion and boosts immune function by raising levels of infection-fighting T-cells (disease-fighting proteins called Gamma-interferon and B-cells), which produce disease-destroying antibodies. Laughter also triggers the release of endorphins, the body's natural painkillers producing a general sense of well-being.

In March of 1995 Dr. Madan Kataria, a family physician from Mumbai, India, decided to write an article called "Laughter - the best medicine" for his monthly health magazine, *My Family Doctor*. He discovered scientific literature that described in great length the proven benefits of laughter on the human mind and body. He decided to test the impact of laughter on himself. The following morning he went to his local public park and somehow managed to convince four people to join him in a "Laughter Club." Within a few days this small group grew to over 50 participants.

Initially they created laughter by telling jokes. Within two weeks, though, the stock of good jokes ran out and it became clear that an alternative had to be found. Dr Kataria re-read all of the scientific research he had on laughter and found that the human mind doesn't make a distinction between fake and genuine laughter. Either way it produced "happy" chemistry. The concept of laughing for no reason was born.

Started initially with just five people in 1995, Dr. Kataria's group has grown into a world-wide movement with more than 5,000 clubs in over 23 countries. Now called "Laughter Yoga," these clubs are usually free of charge. Visit www.laughteryoga.org to find a laughter club near you. Fifteen minutes a day may change your mental and physical state.

Chapter 3

Superfoods for Internal Cleansing

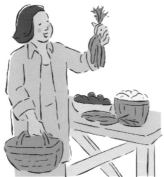

Thirty years ago Americans became afraid to swim in the water for fear of sharks. Now we're afraid to drink the water because of toxins. Just when we summon the courage to get up and face another day, the media sneaks up on us with one more dire report about our toxic environment and its hapless victims. If this trend continues, the boy-in-the-bubble may have lots of company!

On planet Earth we've been exposed to more toxins than any other population in history. Over a lifetime, the average human body has been infiltrated by trans fats, antidepressants, fast food, triple-rich ice cream, recreational drugs, double espressos, alcoholic beverages, antibiotics, second-hand smoke and artificial preservatives too various to name. There's little need to worry about nukes harming us—at this rate, our current lifestyle and environment will get us long before any third-world countries do.

Quick Tip: *So what's a toxin?* A toxin is any substance that irritates or damages our body, putting stress on all our biochemical functions and eroding our health. Because many of the toxins we ingest are stored in fatty tissue, obese people are at a much higher risk for toxicity.

Clean Bits

✓ When a person loses excess weight, they automatically reduce their toxic load. But as these toxins are being released, the body has a much greater need for water, fiber and antioxidants to aid in flushing out the poisons.

✓ Our body handles toxins by neutralizing, transforming or eliminating them.
  o The liver helps transform many toxic substances into harmless agents and also dumps wastes through the bile into the intestines, where much waste is eliminated.
  o The blood carries wastes to the kidneys.
  o We also clear toxins through sweating from exercise or heat.
  o Our sinuses and skin may also be accessory elimination organs whereby excess mucus or toxins can be released, as with sinus congestion or skin rashes.
✓ Anything that supports elimination helps you to detoxify.
✓ Detoxifying your body can give you more energy, sharpen your mental capacity, clear up your complexion and greatly reduce aches and pains.
✓ Many of the most dangerous toxins are fat-soluble, which means that unless they are detoxified they are more likely to lodge in your cells and remain there, causing trouble.
✓ Most of the molecules we create every day are made for the sake of getting rid of waste molecules.

Superfoods for Internal Cleansing

Artichoke

Why: Recent scientific evidence supports the affects of artichoke's active ingredient, cynarin, found in highest concentration in the leaves. Cynarin has significant liver protecting and regenerating effects along with its promoting the flow of bile and fat to and from the liver. Bile is a major player in the detoxification process, as it carries many toxins from the liver to the intestines to be absorbed by fiber and then excreted. Luteolin, a powerful antioxidant found in artichokes, strongly inhibits tumor growth. Also, artichokes have a mild diuretic effect.

Where to buy it: At the grocery store in the produce section.

How much to eat: Eating artichoke once a day is recommended. One medium-sized artichoke provides 54 mg calcium, 72 mg magnesium, 425 mg potassium, folic acid, vitamin K, zinc, copper, manganese and selenium.

Quick Facts: The body makes bile acids from cholesterol. Increased bile acid production results in a decrease in circulating cholesterol. Improved digestion also results from the increased bile flow.

Beets

Why: Beetroot has unique chemicals (e.g. betalains, and betaine) and high levels of important micronutrients. The betalains act as antioxidants. Betaine is a dietary antioxidant with a particularly high bioavailability, with very little being excreted under normal conditions. Just a little beetroot is beneficial. Its other antioxidant nutrients, vitamin C and beta-carotene, help fight infection and help detoxify a range of carcinogenic chemicals. Beetroot stimulates liver, bowel and kidney function, and enhances the elimination of toxins and wastes.

Where to buy it: At the grocery store in the fresh produce section or canned section. Finding fresh beetroot is always the first choice, but consuming canned beets is better than not eating them at all!

How much to eat: A ½ cup is only 37 calories. Make this one of your daily 8 to 10 servings of vegetables and fruits a day, three to four times a week.

Quick Tip:
See Moods and Stress Chapter Two to find out how beets are also a "mood food."

Quick Recipe
Roasted Beet Roots

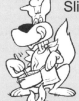

Slice 4 beets about ¼ inch thick.
In a bowl combine:
- ¼ cup extra virgin olive oil
- ½ tsp curry powder
- ¼ tsp sea salt
- ¼ tsp black pepper

Cover the beets with the olive oil mixture and then lay the beets on a baking sheet. Bake in the oven at 380° for 30-40 minutes or until tender.

Cabbage Family Vegetables:
Cabbage, Broccoli and Brussels Sprouts

Why: New research reveals that phytonutrients in the cabbage family actually signal our genes to increase production of enzymes involved in detoxification–the cleansing process through which our body eliminates harmful compounds. The natural synergy that results, optimizes our cells' ability to disarm and clear free radicals and toxins, including potential carcinogens. The chemical sulforaphane, found in these Superfoods, increases the production of antioxidants and detoxification enzymes, both of which eliminate carcinogenic compounds, helping to prevent tumors.

Where to buy it: At the grocery store in the fresh produce section.

How much to eat: Eating one to two servings of any of these three Superfoods daily counts toward your daily 8 to 10 servings of vegetables and fruits as recommended by the FDA.

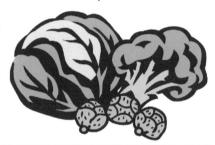

Cereal Grasses:
Barley Grass, Wheat Grass and Alfalfa

Why: Chlorophyll-rich foods, like cereal grasses, lessen the effects of pollutants and pesticides. They help remove drug residues from the body and counter damage from chemical preservatives used in many foods. Using dehydrated, organic cereal grasses such as barley grass, wheat grass and alfalfa as a daily nutritional supplement is a convenient way to add more green foods to your daily diet. These nutrient-dense Superfoods are extremely high in vitamins A, Bs, C, E and K, plus the minerals potassium, selenium, zinc, calcium and phosphorus. They are great antioxidants.

Where to buy it: Health food stores and some progressive grocery stores and drug stores.

How much to eat: You can find these nutrient-dense Superfoods in many Superfood drinks and green drinks. Follow the recommended directions on the package. One serving is recommended for daily use, although if you feel like you need a little more cleansing, take up to three times daily over a shorter period of time (one to two weeks, drinking lots of water).

Quick Facts: Chlorophyll is the molecule that absorbs sunlight and uses its energy to produce carbohydrates from CO_2 and water. This process is known as photosynthesis and is the basis for sustaining the life processes of all plants. Because animals and humans obtain many of their nutrients by eating plants, photosynthesis can be said to be a key source for life.

Quick Tip: In 1780, the famous English chemist Joseph Priestley found that plants could restore air which had been altered by the burning of candles. And in just one summer, a full-grown tree gives off enough oxygen to keep ten humans alive for one full year. Think of trees as giant filters that purify the air we breathe and heal the earth around us.

Cranberries

Why: Cranberry juice acidifies the urine, helping to prevent urinary tract infections. A pathogen must latch on to and then penetrate the mucosal surface of the urinary tract walls for an infection to start; cranberries prevent such adherence. They contain an antibacterial agent called hippuric acid, along with other compounds that reduce the ability of E. coli bacteria to adhere to the walls of the urinary tract. In other words, cranberries detoxify our urinary tract. E. coli is washed away and voided in the urine.

Quick Tip: It's been discovered that the cranberry's proanthocyanidins (antioxidants) are structurally different than the proanthocyanidins found in the other plant foods tested. This explains cranberry's unique, bacterial anti-adhesion activity, helping to maintain urinary tract health.

Where to buy it: At the grocery store as frozen cranberries, frozen juice or as ready-made juice.

How much to drink/eat: Drinking as little as ¼ ounce has proven beneficial; a recommended amount is a six ounce serving daily. You can also add frozen cranberries to your morning or afternoon shake or in a Superfood drink.

Quick Facts: Laboratory studies published in the October 2004 issue of the *Journal of Science, Food and Agriculture* reports that a phytonutrient found in cranberries is effective against herpes simplex virus (HSV-2), the cause of genital herpes. In a manner similar to the way the properties in cranberries protect against bladder infection by preventing bacteria from adhering to the bladder wall, cranberries' antiviral compound, proanthocyanidin A-1, inhibits the attachment and penetration of the herpes virus.

Dandelion Leaves

Why: The bitter compounds in the leaves and root help stimulate digestion and serve as a mild laxative. They also increase bile production in the gall bladder and bile flow from the liver, essential in helping us utilize food nutrients and eliminate waste. The increase in bile flow improves fat (including cholesterol) metabolism in the body. Dandelion is a source of potassium, sodium, calcium, phosphorus and iron. The leaves are a rich source of vitamins A, B, C and D. Dandelions are also a remarkable source of natural potassium, and offer all the advantages of a balanced diuretic in a natural form. It's known as a hepatic herb–an herb, usually bitter, which works particularly well on the liver by toning, nourishing and strengthening it (the liver is the primary blood-cleansing organ of the body).

Where to buy it: Many forward-thinking grocery stores carry dandelion leaves in the fresh produce section. You can also purchase dandelion leaves in a capsule form at health food stores, and it's often an ingredient in Superfood drinks. Dried dandelion leaves, ordered from www.mountainrose.com, make an excellent tea.

How much to eat/drink: Counting this incredible Superfood as one of your daily 8 to 10 servings of vegetables and fruits is great for extra liver protection and digestion aid. Fresh leaves may be added to salads or juiced (the juice extraction is the most potent for medicinal purposes). The dried leaf makes a great-tasting tea and is used as a mild laxative to relieve constipation.

 Quick Tip: Many herbalists view the dandelion as an effective treatment for liver disease, even in extreme cases such as cirrhosis. It can also benefit the pancreas, kidneys, stomach and spleen.

Grapefruit and Lemons

Why: Both are powerful liver protectors, and are known citrus bioflavonoids, antioxidants known to protect against cancers. Grapefruit and lemons both have D-Limone, an antioxidant that promotes the formation of detoxifying enzymes by helping to make toxic chemicals in the liver more water-soluble and therefore more easily excreted from the body. Grapefruit also contain a chemical compound, glucarates, thought to help rid the body of excess estrogen.

Where to buy it: At the grocery store in the fresh produce section.

How much to eat: Add a slice of lemon or grapefruit to your water to enjoy their benefits. One whole lemon or grapefruit daily gives added liver protection and detoxifying enzymes.

Sea Vegetables:
Nova Scotia dulse, Kelp, Arame, Wakame, Kombu and Hijiki

Why: Sea vegetables contain sodium alginate that protects against radiation, environmental pollutants and some heavy metals by binding to toxins and excreting them through the feces. Agar, derived from the sodium alginate in kelp, is a safe, non-toxic substance that can be used as a thickening agent or gelatin and helps cleanse the body.

Where to buy it: Asian markets and some health food stores. Sea vegetables are sold in different forms. Look for sea vegetables sold in tightly-sealed packages. Avoid those showing evidence of excessive moisture. Agar can be found in the baking section of Asian markets.

How much to eat: Eat 4 to 4½ cups fresh or dehydrated sea vegetables a week. Substitute agar for corn starch when thickening sauces during cooking.

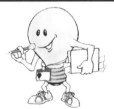

Quick Tip: There are thousands of sea vegetable types, each classified into categories by color, known either as brown, red or green sea vegetables. Each is unique, with a distinct shape, taste and texture. Some of the most popular types:

- **Nori:** (no·ri) Dark purple-black vegetable that turns phosphorescent green when toasted; famous for its role in making sushi rolls.
- **Kelp:** Light brown to dark green in color—often available in flake form. Kelp is nature's richest source of iodine, a component of the thyroid hormones thyroxine (T4) and triiodothyronine (T3).
- **Hijiki:** (hi·ji·ki) Looks like small strands of black, wiry pasta with a strong flavor.
- **Kombu:** (kom·bu) Very dark in color and generally sold in strips or sheets; often used as a flavoring for soups.
- **Wakame:** (wa·ka·me) Similar to kombu, most commonly used to make Japanese miso soup.
- **Arame:** (ar·a·me) This lacy, wiry sea vegetable is sweeter and milder in taste than many others.
- **Dulse:** Soft, chewy texture and reddish-brown in color.

Water, Water, Water

Why: Simply put, drinking water helps dilute and eliminate toxin accumulations. It is likely the most important detoxifier. It helps clean us through our skin and kidneys, and it improves our sweating with exercise. Water also plays an important part during elimination through our colon.

Where to buy it: At the grocery store. Drinking most any type of water is good; the main thing is to drink it. And when you are doing a more intense detoxifying program, drink lots more!

How much to drink: Drink at least ½ your body weight in ounces daily, i.e., 150 pounds divided in half = 75 pounds; next, convert that to ounces = 75 ounces/day. A medium sized bottle of water is approximately 25 ounces. So you should drink **three** of those each day, or drink more!

Quick Facts: Dr. Batmanghelidj in his report, "Medical Report: A New Medical Discovery", states, "Every function inside the body is regulated by and depends on water. Water must be available to carry vital elements, oxygen, hormones and chemical messengers to all parts of the body. Without sufficient water to wet all parts equally, some more remote parts of the body will not receive the vital elements that water supplies."

Herbs for Cleansing

Milk Thistle

Why: The herb, milk thistle, is the subject of several scientific studies suggesting its active substances (particularly silymarin) protect the liver from damage caused by viruses, toxins, alcohol and certain drugs such as acetaminophen. It's known to stimulate production of new liver cells, replacing old, damaged ones. Milk thistle removes excessive iron from the body and promotes bile flow. The active chemical component in the herb is silymarin, which functions 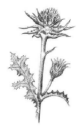 as an antioxidant and is one of the most potent liver protective agents known. Clinical trials have proven silymarin to be effective in treating chronic liver diseases and in protecting the liver from toxic chemicals.

Where to buy it: Health food stores and some drug stores; it's also found in many green drink formulas.

How much to take/eat: As a daily tonic, take 35 mg to 80 mg. To cleanse the liver, take 200 mg, three times a day for only one week. Most milk thistle supplements are a standardized extract (concentrated) that contains 70% - 80% of silymarin.

 Quick Tip: One animal study found that silymarin (the active compound in milk thistle) worked as effectively as the cholesterol-lowering drug, Probucol, with the additional benefit of substantially increasing HDL ("good") cholesterol.

—————— Nutrients for Internal Cleansing ——————

The chemical reactions that take place when the body detoxifies require various vitamins and nutrients:

Vitamin A

Vitamin A helps prevent penetration of toxins by strengthening the walls of cells and lessens the effects of chemical toxins such as medications and pesticides. It's also been found to help counteract ionizing gamma radiation.

Vitamin B1 *(thiamin)*

A powerful antioxidant, vitamin B enhances the performance of the liver.

Vitamin B2 *(riboflavin)*

B2 protects against chemical toxins by activating the antioxidant glutathione (protects cells from oxidative damage).

Vitamin B3 *(niacin)*

B3 helps recycle glutathione in the body. Glutathione detoxifies many chemicals in our body.

Vitamin B6 *(pyridoxine)*

Along with folic acid and B12, B6 detoxifies excess homocysteine caused by high protein diets.

Vitamin B12 *(cobalamin)*

B12 aids in the detoxification of fat-soluble toxic chemicals, lessens the reactions of sulfite preservatives found in foods, helps clear excess estrogen and enhances the flow of bile.

Vitamin C *(ascorbic acid)*

Vitamin C helps counteract the effects of chemical toxins, radiation and reduces the levels of lead in the blood.

Vitamin E *(tocopherol)*

Vitamin E is a powerful antioxidant found to lessen radiation damage, guard against carbon monoxide, chlorine, cigarette smoke, mercury, nitrates and ozone.

Folic Acid

Folic Acid, along with B6 and B12, help with the elimination of excess homocysteine.

Choline

An antioxidant that when taken in the lecithin form, significantly thins bile helping to increase the removal of toxins from the liver. It also helps protect the liver.

Inositol

Supports fat metabolism, helping detoxify toxins found in body fat.

Calcium

Calcium protects against lead toxicity and other metals such as mercury and aluminum. It also supports kidney function (important for blood cleansing).

Magnesium

Detoxifying heavy metals and pesticides, magnesium supports our liver in the detoxification process.

Manganese

Manganese assists in chelation of heavy metals, sulfites and helps eliminate excess iron.

Potassium

Potassium supports detoxification of the kidneys and cleanses the body of excess mercury.

Selenium

Essential for glutathione production, selenium binds with toxic metals so they can be excreted from the body.

Silica

Silica detoxifies aluminum from the body.

Zinc

Zinc provides protection from arsenic, cadmium and mercury in the kidneys.

————— **The Body's Cleansing Systems** —————

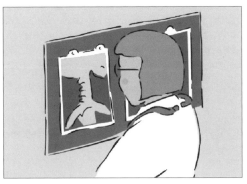

The Digestive System

Processes the foods we consume and identifies toxins for elimination. The liver is the body's most essential cleansing organ. It filters many toxins out of the blood and sends them along in the bile to be removed in feces. The liver processes the toxins where they actually have a chemical transformation. The toxins processed in the liver include bacteria, pesticides found in food, medications and alcohol. Our daily bowel movements are one of the most obvious reminders of our body's continual detoxifying processes. Fat soluble toxins that have traveled out of the liver in bile are then excreted through bowel movements. Signs that may be associated with toxicity in the digestive system are constipation, diarrhea, bloating, gas, yeast, indigestion, allergies, headaches, obesity and fatigue.
(*Learn more about the digestive system in Chapter 4: Superfoods for Digestion and Elimination.*)

The Endocrine System

Regulates the metabolism of the body; when this system is functioning well, toxins are removed more efficiently.

The Lymphatic System

Drains and filters fluids as it detects and removes bacteria. Lymph fluid circulates through the system, coming from the blood and returning to the blood. In this way, the lymphatic fluid not only nourishes vital organs but also removes harmful substances from the body. There are over 600 lymph nodes along our blood vessels throughout our body. Its movement must be supported and enhanced through exercise, hydrotherapy and skin brushing.

The Respiratory System

With every breath, we take in oxygen-rich air through our nose and mouth and our lungs fill up and empty out. And even if the air we breathe is dirty or polluted, our respiratory system can defend itself against foreign matter and organisms that enter through the nose and mouth. Pollutants are breathed out again, coughed up, swallowed, passed out through the intestines or destroyed by digestive juices, or eaten by macrophages, a type of blood cell that patrols the body looking for germs to destroy. Respiration also helps to oxygenate the cells giving nourishment to them so they can do their individual detoxifying tasks.

The Skin

Eliminates fat soluble toxins through the sebaceous glands. When detoxification is not efficient in our other systems, toxins can exit through the skin causing rashes, acne and other conditions. Toxins that use the skin for elimination include DDT and heavy metals such as lead, aluminum and mercury.

The Urinary System

Including the kidneys, bladder, ureters and urethra are one of the main exit routes for toxins. The primary function of the kidney is to filter wastes from our blood. About 50 gallons of blood enter our kidneys every day. The wastes that are filtered and extra water turn into urine. The urine then travels down tubes, called ureters and is stored in the bladder until excretion (urination). Many toxins are made water-soluble by the liver before reaching the kidneys for further filtering and then eliminated in the urine. Difficulty urinating, water retention, low back pain and kidney stones may be signs of toxicity.

The Meaning of Antioxidants

For about 20 years, we've known that many phytonutrients work as "antioxidants" to disarm free radicals before they can damage DNA, cell membranes and fat-containing molecules (such as cholesterol). Most people know the word "antioxidant," but few know what it really means. So here is a simple explanation:

We all know that we need oxygen to live. Oxidation is the process by which we are continuously burning calories to produce energy for our cells to use in order to function. Scientists now know that this very process which enables us to live also releases dangerous and highly-active molecules known as free radicals.

Free radicals are highly-reactive chemicals that attack molecules by capturing electrons and modifying their chemical structures. These free radicals want to attach to something very quickly. If they don't attach to antioxidants (provided through our diet), they attach to another molecule and can produce degenerative change in our bodies. Over a long period of time, such damage can become irreversible, leading to chronic diseases such as cancer, heart disease, Alzheimer's, Parkinson's, rheumatoid arthritis, atherosclerosis and other diseases associated with aging.

An antioxidant is **any** substance that reduces oxidative damage (damage due to oxidation) like that caused by free radicals. The more antioxidants we have in our system, the faster the free radicals can be safely deactivated. It is the job of the antioxidant to keep free radicals from turning healthy molecules into unhealthy molecules. In addition, antioxidants have properties that enable them to repair damage. Antioxidants, like vitamin E, are often added to products to prevent or delay their deterioration when exposed to air.

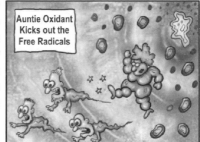

Auntie Oxidant Kicks out the Free Radicals

─────── Cleansing the Phytonutrients Way ───────

Scientists have discovered that it's the combination of phytonutrients that give us the health benefits. In the December 2004 issue of *Journal of Nutrition*, it was said that the actions of antioxidant nutrients alone do not explain the observed health benefits of diets rich in fruits and vegetables, because taken alone, the individual antioxidants studied in clinical trials do not appear to have consistent preventive effects. Studies have shown that fruits and vegetable phytonutrients extracts exhibit strong antioxidants activities from the combinations of phytonutrients. It's the synergistic effects of phytonutrients in fruits and vegetables that attributed to the complex mixture found in whole foods.

Plant foods contain a variety of chemicals, called phytonutrients that improve overall health as well as prevent disease. They help block carcinogens, carry them out of the body, detoxify environmental pollutants and boost the immune system. There are over 12,000 identified phytonutrients; many are antioxidants. Here is a list, grouping phytonutrients into categories based on their structure and content.

Carotenoids *(CAR•ot•uh•noids)*

Why: These are powerful antioxidants that are anti-cancer agents, artery plaque reducers and immune system boosters, often found in brightly-colored vegetables and fruits.

Which foods have it: Carrots, sweet potatoes, yellow squash, tomato, spinach, broccoli, parsley, apricot, mango, papaya, cantaloupe, peaches and mushrooms.

Catechins *(KAT•i•chins)*

Why: These antioxidants are virus and bacterial fighters, anti-cancer agents, a digestion aid and a harmful fat and oil neutralizer.

Which foods have it: Berries, green and black tea.

Flavonoids *(FLAV•uh•noids)*

Why: These antioxidants prevent cancer-causing hormones from attaching to body cells. They protect the eyes and nerves and help with symptoms of allergies, arthritis and asthma.

Which foods have it: Chocolate, citrus fruits, berries, apples, tea, carrots, peppers, cabbage, tomato, squash, eggplant, broccoli, cucumbers, onions, parsley, soybeans and soy products.

Indoles *(in•DOLS)*

Why: Help stimulate the production of detoxifying enzymes, attach to chemical carcinogens making them harmless, protect against cancer and increase the body's detoxification functions.

Which foods have it: Cabbage, cauliflower, broccoli, Brussels sprouts, kale, collard greens, mustard greens and turnips.

Isoflavone *(I•SO•fla•VONES)*

Why: Classified under the antioxidants, bioflavonoids, soy isoflavones are the most studied. They're converted into phytoestrogens in the body, slowing bone degeneration. They're also known to reduce the risk of breast cancer and have cardiovascular health benefits.

Which foods have it: Soybeans and green peas.

Isothiocyanates *(I•SO•thi•o•cy•a•NATES)*

Why: These powerful stimulators of protective enzymes guard against cell damage from potential carcinogens.

Which foods have it: Peanuts, cabbage, broccoli, watercress, kale, horseradish, radishes, rutabaga and soybeans.

Lignans *(lig•nans)*

Why: These antioxidants help suppress cancer, especially colon cancer. They're also cardiovascular protectors and provide anti-inflammatory properties.

Which foods have it: Figs, strawberries, flaxseed, Brazil nuts, peas, carrots, green beans, potatoes and wheat bran.

Limonene *(lim•oh•NENE)*

Why: These antioxidants are found to protect against cancer. They also help dissolve gallstones.

Which foods have it: Citrus fruit (the white part of the inside peel contains the highest source of limonene), lemon grass and celery.

Lutein *(LOO•teen)*

Why: These antioxidants reduce the risk of macular degeneration–an eye disease eventually causing blindness–and lutein is thought to protect against cancer.

Which foods have it: Kale, chard, spinach, turnip greens, chicory, radicchio, arugula, mustard greens and dandelion.

Luteolin *(LOO•te•o•lin)*

Why: These antioxidants strongly inhibit tumor growth, enhance detoxification and protect the liver.

Which foods have it: Artichoke, beets, rosemary, parsley, thyme, celery, spinach and Brussels sprouts.

Lycopene *(LIKE•oh•peen)*

Why: A subgroup of carotenoids, lycopene antioxidants have been found to lower the risk of prostate, breast, lung, gastrointestinal, cervical, bladder and endometrial cancer cells.

Which foods have it: Cooked tomatoes, pink or red grapefruit, watermelon, guava and persimmons.

Monoterpenes *(mono•ter•pene)*

Why: Offering cancer prevention, these antioxidants also lower heart disease and assist in detoxifying carcinogens.

Which foods have it: Ginger, rosemary, thyme, oregano, citrus fruits and cranberries.

Organosulfur *(or•ga•no•sul•fer)*

Why: These are natural antibiotic and antifungal agents.
Which foods have it: Garlic, onions, chives, leeks, watercress, cauliflower, Brussels sprouts, broccoli and cabbage.

Polyphenol *(poly•phe•nol)*

Why: These antioxidants help prevent blood clotting, help lessen the effects of nitric oxide (free radical), prevent LDL cholesterol from oxidizing and are known for cancer prevention.
Which foods have it: Citrus fruits, berries, green and black tea, red wine, grape seeds, chocolate, apple, rhubarb, cranberries, burdock, figs, cinnamon and ginger.

Quercetin *(kwer•CE•tins)*

Why: Classified under the group flavonoids, these antioxidants are cancer suppressors, powerful protectors against allergic reactions, macular degeneration and cataracts.
Which foods have it: Apples, green and black tea, fennel, onions, dill and tarragon.

Sulforaphane *(sul•for•uh•FANE)*

Why: These are cancer inhibitors and also enhance detoxification.
Which foods have it: Broccoli, cauliflower, Brussels sprouts, kale and turnips.

Sterols *(ste•rol)*

Why: These offer cardiovascular benefits and help lower cholesterol levels.
Which foods have it: Olive oil, olives, avocado, cherries, rice bran, rice bran oil, peanuts, alfalfa sprouts, mushrooms, buckwheat, sunflower seeds and pumpkin seeds.

Triterpene *(tri•ter•pin•ese)*

Why: These prevent and fight cancer.
Which foods have it: Citrus fruits, parsley, olive oil, rice bran oil, ginsengs and boswellia.

 Quick Tip: Many baby-boomers just chalk their aching joints up to the aging process. But medical science now says that our lifelong accumulation of toxins can actually be causing extreme fatigue, premature aging, chronic aches and pains, as well as most of our 21st century illnesses.

Exercise

Exercise promotes strong blood circulation and increased flow of lymphatic fluid (the lymphatic system is a major player in detoxifying our body). Exercise stimulates the release of toxins through your skin as you sweat and promotes greater detoxification through the lungs as well as better oxygenation to the cells. Exercise improves the liver detoxification process, and reduces fat reserves where toxins are stored. Exercising as little as 10 minutes, three times a day will help rid the body of waste and toxins.

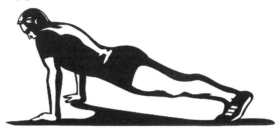

Let Food be Your Medicine

The human body is dependent on nature for both health and wellness. There is evidence of the use of herbal and plant remedies going back some 60,000 years. All cultures have folk medicine histories that include the use of plants and foods. Even in ancient cultures, people methodically and scientifically collected information on plants and foods, developing well-defined natural health remedies.

Herbal medicine goes one step further. It studies the nutrients found in specific herbs that help our bodies holistically repair themselves. Well into the 20th century, much of the pharmacopoeia of scientific medicine was derived from the herbal lore of native peoples. Many drugs are of plant origin. About one-quarter of the prescription drugs dispensed by community pharmacies in the United States contain at least one active ingredient derived from plant material.

As medicine evolved in the United States, plants and food persevered as a mainstay of country medicine. Approaches to natural healing passed from physician to physician, and family to family. There was a partnership between home folk medicine and the family doctor. Physicians often used food, plants and herbal preparations to treat common ills. Many textbooks characterizing plants as proven-by-use prescription medicines were available, offering hundreds of medically useful comments on plant's barks, roots, berries, leaves, resins, twigs and flowers.

As 20th-century technology advanced, simple plant-and-water remedies were gradually discarded. Today, we rely on medications to make us feel better and fight disease instead of eating fresh, healthy foods found in the local grocery store. Giving your body the nutrients it needs to help you fight disease and keep you healthy is the key to living a longer, healthier life. Adding Superfoods to your daily diet is one way to keep you away from the doctor's waiting room. Exercising regularly is also important. Developing a lifestyle that incorporates body-mind-spirit can actually change your life in less than eight weeks!

Chapter 4

· ·

Superfoods for Digestion and Elimination

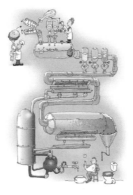

There are countless reports about the relationship between good digestive health and longevity. It's estimated that over a third of the American population suffers from digestion disorders and over $2 billion dollars are spent annually on digestive aids! Keeping your digestive system well tuned, lubricated and moving along is vital to overall good health. If what you put in your mouth is of good quality, then all will exit well at the other end. There are Superfoods to move things regularly, protect our stomach lining, protect against bacteria harmful to our stomach and actually help heal our intestinal lining. Stocking your cupboard with these Superfoods will help you avoid embarrassing situations, frustration in the bathroom or maybe even a health crisis.

Quick Bits

- ✓ Our bodies produce one liter of saliva a day.
- ✓ Every day 11.5 liters (20 pints) of digested food, liquids and digestive juices flow through the digestive system, but only 100 mls (one sixth of a pint) is excreted in feces.
- ✓ Muscles contract in waves to move the food down the esophagus. This means that food would still get to your stomach, even if you stood on your head.
- ✓ Most of feces are made up of fiber which cannot be digested. Fiber gives your food bulk to keep your digestive system moving.

✓ The small intestine is where over 90 percent of digestion and absorption takes place.
✓ The gall bladder stores bile used to break down dietary fat.
✓ The pancreas produces digestive juices and helps control blood sugar.

Superfoods for Digestion and Elimination

Aloe Vera Juice

Why: An herbal bitter which helps gastric juices flow, aloe vera contains protein, calcium, magnesium, zinc, vitamins A, C, and E, vitamin B-complex; and essential fatty acids–all valuable components of a healthy diet. This gel contains carbohydrate polymers that helps heal the stomach, ease constipation and prevent continuing diarrhea, giving regularity to the bowels. Aloe vera is increasingly popular in the treatment of Irritable Bowel Syndrome (IBS) and associated digestive problems.

Where to buy it: Most health food stores and some drug stores carry a good high quality aloe vera juice suitable for internal use.

How much to take: Recommended dose is 1 tablespoon in water before each meal.

Angostura Bitters *(an·guh·STOOR·eh)*

Why: Angostura bitters is made of herbs and spices. The main ingredient is gentian. Gentian extract stimulates the appetite, stimulates the secretion of saliva and gastric juices, and accelerates the emptying of the stomach. Gentian root also stimulates the gallbladder, pancreas and mucous membranes of the stomach, thus contributing to an increased secretion of digestive juices and enzymes.

Where to buy it: Angostura bitters is usually sold anywhere that liquor is sold. Be aware that the alcohol content is 45% by volume.

How much to take/eat: Gentian preparations, like Angostura Bitters, are most effective if taken 30 minutes before mealtime. Its activity begins about five minutes after reaching the stomach, as digestive juices begin to flow and the secretion of bile increases. This provides for better digestion of fats and proteins.

Bananas

Why: Known for their antacid effects, bananas protect against stomach ulcers and ulcer damage by activating the cells that compose the stomach lining, producing a thicker protective mucus barrier against stomach acids. Bananas also help eliminate bacteria in the stomach, pinpointed as a primary cause of stomach ulcers. Bananas contain pectin, a soluble fiber that helps normalize movement through the digestive tract and ease constipation.

Where to buy it: At the grocery store.

How much to eat: Bananas have a high sugar content (+60 glycemic index for a ripe banana). Less ripe bananas have a lower GI number of 30 (below 50 is considered low). If you aren't worried about high blood sugar levels, eating ½ a banana per day will help heal your stomach.

Barley-Grain

Why: Barley is a great way to provide consistent bulk to your digestive tract. It also helps decrease the transit time of fecal matter, decreasing the risk of colon cancer and hemorrhoids. Barley's dietary fiber provides food for the "friendly" bacteria in the large intestine (not all grains do this). Friendly bacteria protects the intestinal tract from pathogenic (disease-causing) bacteria. The fiber in barley can also help to prevent blood sugar levels from rising too high in people with diabetes. For Irritable Bowel Syndrome sufferers, barley's fiber can add bulk to the stool, thereby reducing the discomfort of either diarrhea or constipation.

Where to buy it: At the grocery store in the dried bean and grain section.

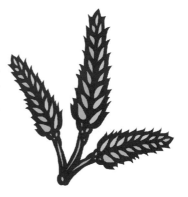

How much to eat: Eat ½ cup of barley or combine it with ½ cup of wheat, oat or rice bran daily to keep you regular. Cook 1 cup barley to 3 cups liquid; bring to a boil; then simmer on lower heat and cover for approximately 45 minutes to an hour.

Quick Recipe
Barley and Wild Rice Pilaf with Pomegranate Seeds

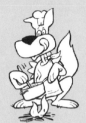

- 2 tsp extra-virgin olive oil
- 1 medium onion, finely chopped
- ½ cup wild rice, rinsed
- ½ cup pearl barley
- 3 cups reduced-sodium chicken broth or vegetable broth
- ⅓ cup pine nuts
- 1 cup pomegranate seeds
- 2 tsp freshly grated lemon zest, preferably organic
- 2 Tbls chopped fresh flat-leaf parsley

Heat oil in a large saucepan over a medium heat. Add onion and cook, stirring often, until soft. Add wild rice and barley; stir for a few seconds. Add chicken broth and bring to a simmer. Reduce heat to low, cover and simmer until the wild rice and barley are tender and most of the liquid has been absorbed, about 45 to 50 minutes. Toast pine nuts in a small, dry skillet over medium-low heat, stirring constantly, until light golden and fragrant, 2 to 3 minutes. Transfer to a small bowl to cool. Add pomegranate seeds, lemon zest, parsley and toasted pine nuts to the pilaf; fluff with a fork. Serve hot.

Bitter Greens:
Dandelion, Arugula (ah•ROO•guh•lah) chicory, radicchio and endive

Why: Eating a salad of dandelion, arugula, chicory, radicchio and endive will help get your gastric juices flowing. They are all considered bitter greens, yet have a great taste. If you want a mixture of less bitter greens, add some fresh baby greens, such as spinach and a variety of lettuce leaves to the mix.

    ✓ **Dandelion Leaves.** Dandelion is a common meadow herb related to the sunflower family and chicory plant. Dandelion is a great source of potassium, sodium, calcium, phosphorus and iron. The leaves are a richer source of vitamin A than carrots and contain vitamins B, C and D. The bitter compounds help stimulate digestion. They also increase bile production in the liver and bile flow from the gallbladder. The increase in bile flow can help improve fat metabolism, including cholesterol.

✓ **Arugula.** Arugula is also referred to as rucola, roquette and rocket. It's also mildly bitter with a peppery taste. It resembles radish leaves.

✓ **Chicory.** Chicory is cultivated and used as endive under the common names **radicchio, Belgian endive** and **French endive**. It's grown in complete darkness to keep new leaves tender and pale. It has a slightly bitter taste.

Where to buy it: In the produce section of your grocery store. Many packaged, pre-mixed baby greens can be found at most supermarkets. They contain a mixture of some bitter greens.

How much to eat: Eating a bowl full (about 1-2 cups) before the entrée will help your body create the enzymes needed to digest your meal.

Cabbage

Why: Raw cabbage juice is well documented as being remarkably effective in treating peptic ulcers. In one study, one liter of the fresh juice per day (taken in divided doses) resulted in total ulcer healing in an average of ten days. The high content of glutamine is likely the reason for cabbage juice's efficacy in healing ulcers. Glutamine is the major fuel for cells–and helps repair the lining–in the small intestine.

Where to buy it: The fresh produce section of your grocery store.

How much to eat/drink: A ½ cup to 1 cup daily provides one of the 8 to 10 recommended daily servings of vegetables and fruits. One liter per day of the fresh juice, taken in divided doses, may result in total ulcer healing in an average of only 10 days.

Quick Facts: Research has focused on the beneficial phytochemicals in cabbage, particularly its indole-3-carbinole (I3C), sulforaphane and indoles. These compounds help activate and stabilize the body's antioxidant and detoxification mechanisms that dismantle and eliminate cancer-producing substances helping prevent colon cancer.

Cardamom Seeds

Why: Cardamom seeds contain large amounts of oil that stimulates digestion, relieves discomfort from flatulence and counteracts acidity of the stomach. It is the richest known source of the compound cineole, a potent antiseptic that kills bad breath bacteria. The seeds have a slightly lemon flavor and scent.

Where to buy it: You can buy cardamom in three forms: the green whole pods, decorticated (just the small black seeds in the pod) and ground. Cardamom is in most markets, natural food stores and Indian markets. It's one of the more expensive spices, and you will most likely get the best price in the Indian markets.

How much to eat: Instead of carrying around breath mints and stomach acids, carry a small container of cardamom seeds. Five to six seeds chewed well will help relieve gas, indigestion and bad breath. It's also great as a tea alone or in a tea blend.

 Quick Tip: For indigestion, place 15 ground seeds in ½ cup of hot water with ½ teaspoon fresh or dried ginger root and one cinnamon stick. Simmer over low heat for 15 minutes, then add ½ cup of milk and simmer 10 more minute. Add two to three drops of vanilla and then sweeten with honey. Drink one to two cups daily.

Ginger

Why: Ginger is very effective in alleviating symptoms of gastrointestinal distress. In herbal medicine, ginger is regarded as an excellent carminative (promotes the elimination of intestinal gas) and intestinal spasmodic (relaxes and soothes the intestinal tract). It's also a great antioxidant and has very effective anti-inflammatory properties. Whenever possible, choose fresh ginger over the dried form; it will taste better and contain higher levels of gingerol and protease (an anti-inflammatory compound).

Where to buy it: At the grocery store in the fresh produce section.

How much to eat: You can eat ginger daily to soothe your stomach. Make a tea from the fresh roots. Thinly slice the root, add 1 teaspoon to 1 cup water, bring to a boil and let simmer for 10 to 15 minutes. You can always make more and put it in the refrigerator—it's wonderful as a cold drink.

 Quick Tip: If you have a juicer, juice ginger and put it into ice cube trays, place in the freezer and add them to your daily green drink.

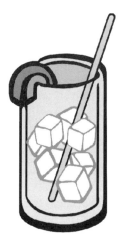

Papaya

Why: Contains the digestive enzyme, papain, an enzyme which helps to digest protein in food. It's a rich source of antioxidant nutrients such as carotenes, vitamin C and flavonoids; the B vitamins, folate and pantothenic acid; and the minerals, potassium and magnesium and fiber. Together, these nutrients promote the health of the cardiovascular system and also provide protection against colon cancer. If you suffer from celiac disease (cannot digest wheat proteins) adding papaya to your diet can help you tolerate these proteins better.

Where to buy it: The fresh produce section of the grocery store.

How much to eat: ½ cup to 1 cup daily counts as one of your 8 to 10 daily servings of vegetables and fruits. Add a squeeze of lemon juice over the papaya for added digestion comfort.

Quick Facts: Papain also exhibits pain relieving properties and the FDA has approved its medicinal use to ease the discomfort of slipped discs (prolapsed inter vertebral disc). Papain is injected into herniated inter vertebral lumbar discs to relieve pain caused by pressure on nerves.

Peppermint Leaves

Why: It calms the muscles of the stomach and improves the flow of bile, which the body uses to digest fats, aiding food to pass through the stomach more quickly. Peppermint leaves can help you get rid of painful digestive gas.

Quick Facts: A number of studies have shown the beneficial effects of enteric-coated peppermint capsules for treating symptoms of IBS, such as pain, bloating, gas and diarrhea. Enteric-coated capsules keep the oil from being released in the stomach, which can lead to heartburn and indigestion.

Where to buy it: Many grocery stores carry peppermint leaves in the fresh produce section. Peppermint is easy to grow; it's a wonderful perennial that comes back faithfully year after year. Because it's so hardy, you may want to grow it in a container to keep it from spreading. You can also purchase dried peppermint leaves at many herb shops.

How much to eat: Adding ¼ cup of peppermint leaves to your bitter salad will help break up the bitterness of the greens. Also drinking peppermint tea before or after dinner helps settle the stomach. As a tea, pour 1 cup of boiling water over 1 to 2 teaspoons of dried leaf and steep for ten minutes.

 Quick Tip: Combining dried peppermint leaves, ginger and green tea together as a digestive herbal cocktail to drink after a meal will help settle your stomach and give you added antioxidant protection.

Pineapple

Why: Fresh pineapple is rich in bromelain, a group of sulfur-containing proteolytic (protein-digesting) enzymes that not only aid digestion, but can effectively reduce inflammation and swelling. Pineapple is a good source of manganese and contains significant amounts of vitamin C and vitamin B1.

Where to buy it: The fresh produce section of your grocery store. You can also find bromelain in vitamin shops and health food stores in capsule or powder form.

How much to eat: Add ½ cup fresh pineapple as one of your 8 to 10 servings of vegetables of fruits if you have digestive discomfort. Pineapple can be acidic for some people. Eating ¼ cup should do the trick.

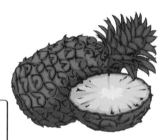

 Quick Tip: As an anti-inflammatory, eat pineapple alone between meals.

Turmeric

Why: The yellow or orange pigment of turmeric, which is called curcumin, is thought to be the primary pharmacological agent in turmeric. Turmeric aids digestion, promotes absorption and regulates metabolism. It's a powerful medicine that has long been used in the Chinese and Indian systems of medicine as an anti-inflammatory agent to treat a wide variety of conditions, including flatulence, jaundice, and colic. It has a soothing and bolstering effect on the mucosa of the gut, boosts stomach defenses against excess acid, drugs and other irritating substances ingested. Turmeric stimulates the flow of bile, protecting against damage from toxins and improving the metabolism of fats.

Where to buy it: The grocery store or Indian market.

How much to eat: ¼ to ½ teaspoon (one quarter to one half) of the powder in a tea two to three times daily between meals. To make the tea, place ½ teaspoon of powder to one cup of boiling water, infuse for five minutes, strain and drink. You can add ginger or cardamom to add flavor.

 Quick Tip: Turmeric can be taken in capsules as a supplement. Take 250-500 mg three times daily. Combining turmeric with bromelain enhances its absorption.

Water–of course!

Why: Drinking liquids with meals is a matter of preference, although there's no clear evidence it helps with digestion. The stomach needs water to digest foods, but it draws in what it needs from the rest of the body.

Water helps prevent constipation by adding more liquid and keeping things moving on through your system. It assists your intestines to do their job more efficiently by keeping things moist. Constipation is a sign that you're not moving your bowels enough, and if your bowel movements are hard and dry, they can't get through your large intestine.

Where to buy it: This fantastic elixir of life can be found in your very own home. Or if you're on the move, all stores carry bottled water.

How much to drink: Drink at least ½ your body weight in ounces, i.e., 150 pounds divided in half = 75 pounds; next, convert that to ounces = 75 ounces/day. A medium sized bottle of water is approximately 25 ounces. So you should drink **three** of those each day.

—— Nutrients for Digestion and Elimination ——

Vitamin A

Vital to the health of the intestinal mucosa, without sufficient vitamin A the mucous membranes become hardened and are more easily penetrated, leading to "leaky gut," ulceration and irritable bowel syndrome. It has been used successfully to treat gastritis and peptic ulcers.

71

Vitamin B3 *(niacin)*

Digestive problems such as bloating, abdominal distention or pain, heartburn and belching are often caused by a lack of stomach acid (hypochlorhydria). Hypochlorhydria can be traced to a relative lack of vitamin B3. Some people have higher than normal requirements for vitamin B3, especially when under stress. If this need isn't met then digestive problems can arise.

Vitamin B5

Vitamin B5 helps alleviate constipation by stimulating peristalsis in the intestinal tract. It's also been found to help with hydrochloric acid production.

Vitamin C

Vitamin C contributes to the health of all the epithelial cells as well as the integrity of the blood vessels that nourish the intestinal tract.

Vitamin E

Needed for muscle tone and a healthy nervous system, a vitamin E deficiency has also been linked to digestive problems such as peptic ulcers, colitis and cancer of the colon.

Protein

Protein is necessary for the maintenance of the mucous membrane in the stomach, particularly the amino acids cystine, lysine and arginine. It's thought that arginine may also increase blood circulation to the stomach, help prevent gastric ulcers, inhibit the ability of alcohol to cause gastric ulcers and improve the function of the kidneys.

Glutamine

An amino acid, glutamine may help prevent gastric ulcers and accelerate their healing. It increases the blood circulation to the stomach and helps control the loss of water from the intestines. It is an important function of intestinal nutrient absorption and for kidney health.

Phosphatidylcholine

Studied by German researchers, phosphatidylcholine was found beneficial to the mucosal lining of the digestive tract.

Zinc

Deficiencies of zinc have been associated with Crohn's Disease, as Crohn's suffers are often found to be deficient in zinc. Zinc may help to restore the integrity of the intestines in Crohn's Disease patients and help accelerate the healing of gastric ulcers.

The Guts of it All...

The digestive tract is a long tube of organs including the esophagus, stomach and intestines. Other organs play a part in digestion, such as the liver and pancreas. The digestive tract is between 25–35 feet long, from the beginning (mouth) to the end (anus). Every morsel of food we eat has to be broken down into nutrients that can be absorbed by the body, which is why it takes hours to fully digest food. Whole food is taken in at the mouth and waste is expelled at the end. Along the intestinal route, nutrients are taken out of the food and absorbed into the bloodstream, according to the body's needs. The whole process is called digestion and then elimination. When something goes wrong along the line, it's known as "indigestion."

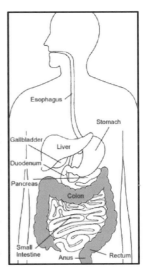

A Bite of Food Begins the Journey

Digestion begins in the brain. Your eyes and your nose put your body and mind in the mood for food. Just the thought of eating food begins the digestive juices flowing. The saliva begins flowing in anticipation of eating; it bathes the first bite with the digestive enzyme, salivary amylase. The amylase enzyme breaks the chemical bonds between the carbohydrate molecules, changing them into smaller sugar molecules. The fat in the food gets a head start on digestion while in the mouth by receiving a tiny squirt of a fat-digesting enzyme called lingual lipase. Chewing helps break the food into smaller particles so the digestive enzymes have easier access to the contents inside.

In the Stomach

The food continues down the esophagus, the tube that connects the mouth and the stomach. The stomach muscles twist and churn the food like a food processor. The lining of the stomach secretes gastric juices, including hydrochloric acid (which dissolves the food), a protein-splitting enzyme called pepsin, and a fat-digesting enzyme called lipase. Glands in the lining of the stomach produce about three quarts of these digestive juices each day. The stomach not only digests, it disinfects. Its hydrochloric acid is strong enough to eat through meat and potent enough to kill most of the harmful bacteria that may be in food. Yet it does not destroy all the bacteria we ingest. Our body requires good bacteria in the large intestine to help maintain our health.

Uh-Oh Indigestion

When the stomach is empty, the lining pours out acid (this can also happen when under stress) and the acid irritates the stomach lining, causing uncomfortable sensations, or indigestion. Adding alcohol or coffee on an empty stomach (accompanied by stress) can literally eat you up inside. Or, the excess acid can squirt up into the esophagus, which has a more sensitive lining, causing "heartburn" or acid reflux.

Quick Tip: Some substances, such as alcohol, salt, caffeine, sugars, water and some drugs (such as aspirin) can be absorbed through the lining of the stomach. This accounts for the blurred speech or the buzz that occurs even before someone finishes his or her glass of wine or cup of coffee. Consuming these substances on an empty stomach increases the speed of their absorption.

Quick Tip: Before you go to the buffet line, visualize the size of your stomach. An average adult's stomach is about 12 inches long and is six inches wide at its widest point. Its capacity is about one quart. Keeping your food intake to less than that size can help with digestion. In fact, research shows that eating four or five small meals a day can help with digestion problems.

On to the Intestine

Most of the consumed proteins and carbs empty from the stomach into the small intestine within a couple hours. Yet the fats remain in the stomach a few hours longer, giving you the feeling of fullness longer after a high fat meal. Digestion continues in the small intestine, absorbing nutrients into the bloodstream. As the food moves down the small intestine it gets squirts of digestive juices that further break down the proteins, carbohydrates and fats into molecules small enough to seep into the bloodstream. Each nutrient requires specific intestinal juices that work on its molecules in particular ways. The pancreas produces enzymes that help digest proteins, fats and carbohydrates. The liver produces bile (stored in the gallbladder) which helps the body absorb fat. The enzymes involved in digestion work on a supply and demand basis. If there's too much food to digest and there's not enough enzymes to process the food, the food gets moved along to the lower intestines where it is not very welcome; indigestion results. Eating smaller meals will save you from discomfort.

The inner wall of the small intestine is covered with millions of microscopic, finger-like projections called villi. These are the transporters of nutrients from the small intestine to the bloodstream. The intestinal lining is only one cell thick allowing nutrients to be easily absorbed. This delicate lining is easily injured by irritants, causing diarrhea, abdominal pain, gas, bloating and auto immune disorders such as allergies and arthritis.

Colon Who?

We're ten hours into our bite of food and it's traveled between 20 and 30 feet and most of its nutrients have been absorbed. The last five feet of the digestive tract is the large intestines or colon. Little digestion occurs in the colon since it has few villi and low levels of intestinal enzymes. However, the colon plays an active and important role in the health and well-being of the whole body. The colon absorbs excess water from the food and provides it to the water-thirsty body. If there isn't enough water in the final waste (broken down food), the colon fills the stool with water to prevent constipation. Healthy water balance in the colon leads to healthy stool patterns.

Also billions of bacteria (intestinal flora) reside in the large intestine. These intestinal bacteria are also known as *probiotics.* The term "probiotics" is also used for bacteria supplements found in many green drinks or in powder or capsule form. The two main healthy bacteria in the colon are lactobacilli and bifidus bacteria. This healthy bacteria keeps the harmful bacteria in check. They also ferment the soluble fiber in food, which nourishes the cells of the large intestine, stimulating healing and reducing the development of intestinal cancer and inhibiting the growth of yeast and disease-causing bacteria. Good bacterium also helps our body make many of our B vitamins.

Oops! Pardon My Gas...

When the normal bacteria living in the large intestines "eat" certain foods (such as beans), the byproduct of the bacteria's own digestive process is gas. While the colon absorbs some of this gas, some goes up and creates bad breath. The rest of the gas is expelled at the other end. This odorous gas is a combination of methane and hydrogen sulfite. Most of the gas you hear, feel or smell is a result of the intestinal bacteria digesting the sugars and fiber that manage to reach the large intestine. How much gas is produced by what foods is very individualized. The amount of food you eat can also cause gas.

Quick Facts: Most of us pass somewhere between 200 and 2,000 ml of gas per day (averaging about 600 ml) in roughly 13 to 14 passages. These emissions are composed of five gasses: nitrogen (N_2), oxygen (O_2), carbon dioxide (CO_2), hydrogen (H_2) and methane (CH_4). Nitrogen usually predominates, followed by variable concentrations of carbon dioxide, hydrogen, methane and very low levels of oxygen. Gas gets into our system by (1) production within the bowel and colon (which accounts for most) and (2) by swallowing air (which accounts for very little). As best we can figure out, most air that is swallowed comes out the way it went in—belched.

The End is Near...

The waste (feces) removal process occurs when the nerves lining the rectum sense the presence of feces that need to be evacuated. It stimulates a reflex causing the muscles of the abdomen and upper rectum to contract and the muscle encircling the anus to relax. This allows easy passage of stool. Eating too little fiber, not drinking enough fluids, eating too much fat (fat slows intestinal transit) and simply not paying attention to the evacuation warnings of the rectum will cause the reflex to stop working, causing constipation.

Chapter 5

Superfoods in Heart Health

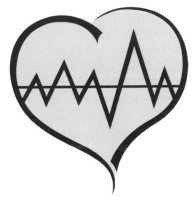

Analogies can get annoying. And sports analogies in business make us want to run for the hills. Things like, "hitting a home run," "going for the gold," or "taking one for the team" are examples of the kinds of statements that over simplify, making us feel like we're living a typical Dilbert comic strip. But analogies can be helpful. So here comes one: gas stations don't sell poor, line-clogging fuel. They know consumers don't want expensive repair bills, but prefer cars that run at peak performance. Poor, artery-clogging foods have the same effect on our bodies. It's a simple analogy but true: heart-healthy food gives the body what it needs to move, think and even rest at peak performance. Healthy eating is how we feed the "engine of our body." So go run for the hills, and when you get back, fill 'er up with premium salads, fruits and lean protein.

> **Quick Facts:** A study published in the *Journal of the American Medical Association* (JAMA) in July 2003 compared a whole foods diet head-to-head with treatment by statin drugs (cholesterol lowering medication). They found a whole foods approach to be so effective that JAMA titled its article, "Diet First, Then Medication for Hypercholesterolemia (High Cholesterol)."

Heart Hits

- ✓ The human heart weighs less than a pound and is the size of your fist
- ✓ **All** the blood in your body cycles through your heart roughly once every minute. In one day, your heart pumps about 2,000 gallons of blood!

✓ The "boomp-boomp" noise your heart makes when it beats is made primarily by the closing of valves during each cycle.

✓ The smaller the animal, the faster its heart beats. For example, a hummingbird has a heart rate of about 1,000 beats per minute and an elephant's heart beats about 25 times per minute. The human heart beats during rest, approximately 60 beats per minute.

✓ The first heart attack was diagnosed in 1912 by James B. Herrick, an American physician.

✓ Place your hand on your heart. Did you place your hand on the left side of your chest? Many people do, but the heart is actually located just about in the center of the chest, between the lungs. It's tipped slightly so a part of it sticks out and taps against the left side of the chest, which is what makes it feel as though it is located there.

✓ Give a tennis ball a good, hard squeeze. You're using about the same amount of force your heart uses to pump blood out to the body. Even at rest, the muscles of the heart work twice as hard as the leg muscles of a sprinter.

✓ The aorta, the largest artery in the body, is about the diameter of a garden hose. Capillaries, on the other hand, are so small that it takes ten of them to equal the thickness of one human hair.

Superfoods for Heart Health

Brown Rice

Why: Brown rice contains magnesium needed for healthy heart muscles, contributing to a nice steady beat. Plus, it's a good source of vitamin B6 (necessary in preventing homocysteine build-up in your blood) and B3 to help lower cholesterol levels. Brown rice also is a good source of iron, selenium and protein.

Quick Fact: Homocysteine can damage blood vessels in several ways, injuring the cells that line arteries and stimulating the growth of smooth muscle cells. It can also disrupt normal blood clotting mechanisms, increasing the risk of clots that can bring on a heart attack or stroke.

Brown Rice Versus White Rice: During the milling and polishing process that converts brown rice into white rice, the nutritional value changes dramatically, destroying 67% of the vitamin B3, 80% of the vitamin B1, 90% of the vitamin B6, 50% of the manganese, 50% of the phosphorus, 60% of the iron, and all of the dietary fiber and essential fatty acids. Fully milled and polished white rice is so lifeless that it requires "enrichment" of vitamins B1, B3 and iron. Brown rice is superior nutritionally to white rice and ought to be your "rice of choice."

Where to buy it: At any grocery store or health food store.

How much to eat: One cup of brown rice combined with vegetables three to four times a week will help protect your heart.

> *Quick Tip 1:* Either short or long grain brown rice is good. Rice is typically cooked with 2 cups water to 1 cup rice. Using a small rice cooker ensures your rice is ready in 25 minutes without stirring!

> *Quick Tip 2:* Combining the following spices to 2 cups rice while cooking will give you extra antioxidant protection:
>
> | | |
> |---|---|
> | ✓ ½ tsp cumin | ✓ ¼ tsp cloves |
> | ✓ ¼ tsp nutmeg | ✓ ¼ tsp ginger |
> | ✓ ¼ tsp cinnamon | ✓ ¼ tsp turmeric |

Cranberries and Blueberries

Why: A study of the *American Chemical Society* released in March, 2003, reported that after drinking three, 6-ounce glasses of cranberry juice per day the subjects' HDL (good) cholesterol increased by an average of 10%. This may seem insignificant, however, it equates to approximately a 40% reduction in heart disease! A compound found in both cranberries and blueberries, called Pterostilbene (PPAR•alpha), is crucial for the metabolism of lipids, including cholesterol. Blueberries are packed with antioxidant phytonutrients called anthocyanidins (ăn'thō•sī'ə•nĭn) which neutralize free radicals. Anthocyanins improve the integrity of the veins and entire vascular system.

Where to buy it: At the grocery store-fresh, dried, frozen or as a juice (with little to no sugar added) are all good sources.

How much to eat/drink: Adding two to three servings (½ cup fresh or 6 ounces of sugar-free juice is a serving) of either cranberries or blueberries can be counted as one of the daily recommended 8 to 10 servings of fruits or vegetables.

Garlic

Why: Studies have verified eating garlic regularly lowers blood pressure, lowers LDL and triglyceride levels, and increases HDL levels. Garlic's beneficial cardiovascular effects are due to not only its sulfur compounds, but its vitamin C, vitamin B6, selenium and manganese content.

Where to buy it: At the grocery store-buying fresh garlic will give you the best heart health results.

How much to eat: Adding at least ½ of a clove of garlic to at least one daily meal is recommended. If you find you just can't handle eating it fresh, or in cooked dishes, consider taking garlic in capsule form. Garlic supplements are found in health food stores and many drug stores. Follow the recommended directions.

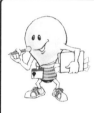

Quick Tip: Despite garlic's many culinary and health benefits, there is one serious drawback: it's hard to prevent garlic breath. Garlic is full of sulphorous compounds. These compounds "feed" the bacteria in the mouth and bad breath (halitosis) results. Unfortunately, you can rarely smell it yourself–although your partner will surely let you know! Try eating a sprig of fresh parsley with your garlic; it won't prevent garlic breath completely, but it helps. Chewing cardamom seeds, found at many Indian markets, can help too.

Quick Facts: A study published in the March, 2006 issue of *Journal of Nutrition* shows that garlic also inhibits coronary artery calcification. In this year-long study, patients given an aged garlic extract daily showed an average increase in their calcium score of 7.5%, while those in the placebo group had an average increase in calcium score of 22.2%.

Grapefruit, Red

Why: When eaten daily, red grapefruit lowered LDL cholesterol levels in 30 days by 15.5% and triglyceride levels lowered by 17.2%, as reported in the March, 2006 *Journal of Agricultural and Food Chemistry*. Additionally, grapefruits significantly improve blood levels of protective antioxidants. Although you get the best heart health results from red grapefruit, other types of grapefruit provide benefits too.

Where to buy it: At the grocery store in the produce section.

How much to eat/drink? Both fresh grapefruit or grapefruit juice will add to heart health. Research shows that drinking a 6 ounce glass of grapefruit juice daily will continue to show 30% of its effectiveness, even after 24 hours.

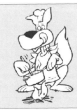

Quick Recipe

Grapefruit can be eaten like an orange. Cut ends, then cut in half and then into slices. If you need to sweeten, add a little honey on the halves.

Quick Tip: Consult your doctor if taking statin medication (prescribed to help lower cholesterol levels). Compounds in grapefruit are known to increase circulating levels of several statin prescription drugs. It may even be possible to lower your dose of medication while increasing your consumption of grapefruit.

Green Tea

Why: Green tea lowers the risk of atherosclerosis by lowering LDL and triglycerides and raising HDL levels. The primary catechin (KAT•uh•kins) in green tea, EGCG (epigallocatechin-3-gallate), prevents heart muscle damage before and after a heart attack and helps thin the blood preventing formation of blood clots.

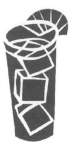

Where to buy it: At the grocery store.

How much to drink: Most studies suggest at least three to four cups (18–24 ounces) a day. The best way to take advantage of green tea's health benefits is to drink it freshly brewed, after steeping the leaves for one to five minutes. Steep the leaves for ten minutes to raise the level of caffeine.

Quick Facts: Reports show the risk of developing high blood pressure was 46% lower among those who drank ½ cup to 2 ½ cups per day, and 65% less among those consuming more than 2 ½ cups per day.

Quick Tip 1: EGCG is the most active component in green tea, and is a stronger antioxidant than either vitamin C or E.

Quick Tip 2: Beware—many products on the market are touting green tea's benefits, but the heart-healthy catechins (found in freshly brewed green tea) are not well absorbed from products like bottled green tea drinks, instant green tea, green tea candy, ice cream and gum. The best benefits are found in freshly-brewed green tea or green tea extracts found in Superfood drinks or capsules.

Lentil Beans

Why: A study published in the *Archives of Internal Medicine* confirms that eating high fiber foods, such as lentils, helps prevent heart disease. Lentils contain significant amounts of folate and magnesium and are a good source of iron, potassium and protein all nutrients that affect heart health by promoting smooth running heart muscles and maintaining low blood pressure.

Where to buy it: At the grocery store.

How much to eat: At least three to five servings a week.

Quick Tip: Lentils are one of the most digestible legumes. Add a few bay leaves to the water while cooking beans for help with digestion. Also add 1 tablespoon of oil to the water to stop foaming. They cook easily and quickly and are great in chili and soups.

Oats, Oat Bran and Oatmeal

Why: Oats, oat bran and oatmeal contain a specific type of fiber known as beta-glucan, which is known to lower cholesterol levels (keeping arteries clear of blockages), which in turn provide necessary nutrients to heart muscles.

Where to buy it: At the grocery store.

How much to eat: About a ½ cup per day. If you like the convenience of instant oatmeal, purchase one that has a small amount of sugar. Look for less than two grams of sugar per serving.

Quick Facts: Studies show that consuming just three grams of soluble oat fiber per day (an amount found in one bowl of oatmeal) typically lowers total cholesterol by 8 to 23% (in people with cholesterol above 220 mg/dl). This is significant because each 1% drop in cholesterol translates to decrease in the risk of developing heart disease by 2%.

Quick Tip: Oatmeal is full of soluble fiber that lowers LDL levels. Experts aren't exactly sure how, but they believe that when you digest fiber, it becomes gooey. Once in your intestines oatmeal sticks to cholesterol and stops it from being absorbed. So instead of absorbing cholesterol into your system—and your arteries—it's simply eliminated as waste.

Quick Facts: In a 2005 study published in the *American Journal of Clinical Nutrition*, researchers tested cholesterol-lowering drugs against cholesterol lowering foods in a group of 34 adults with high cholesterol. Oat products were among the chosen foods. The results were striking: The oat diet lowered cholesterol levels about as well as cholesterol drugs.

Olive Oil

Why: Olive oil, which is high in monounsaturated fat–the "good" fat–combats coronary heart disease by helping to keep HDL cholesterol levels up and LDL cholesterol down. Olive oil also contains phenols, tocopherols (vitamin E) and other natural antioxidants.

Where to buy it: At the grocery store–look for extra virgin olive oil.

How much to eat: Consuming just 1 to 2 tablespoons a day is beneficial. Substitute olive oil for butter when you crave that slice of bread and butter. Add a few drops of balsamic vinegar to the oil for a better taste.

Quick Facts: In a study found in the *Archives of Internal Medicine,* Vol. 160, March 27, 2000: Over one year 23 men and women with mild hypertension were told to add olive oil to their food after cooking, while the other group was asked to add sunflower oil. After six months the average systolic blood pressure in the olive oil group had dropped to 127 mm Hg from the 134 mm Hg recorded at the start and the diastolic pressure had dropped from 90 mm Hg to 84 mm Hg. The level of antihypertensive medication was adjusted during the experiment by a separate group of doctors who did not know which diet their patients were following. The ones in the olive oil group were able to reduce their medication use by an average 48% and eight of them were able to discontinue their medications completely. None of the ones in the sunflower oil group were able to discontinue their medications and the average reduction in medication usage was only 4%.

Quick Tip: Olive oil is the only vegetable oil that can be created simply by pressing the raw material, olives. The quality of the oil depends on the amount of processing involved. Extra virgin olive oil is the least processed and is considered nutritionally best.

Pistachio Nuts

Why: Pistachio nuts are jam-packed with the nutrients needed to provide protection from oxygen damage in the heart muscle, with CoQ10, protein, magnesium, calcium, potassium, vitamin A, E and B vitamins. Plus, they contain a high level of beta-sitosterol (plant sterols), one of several plant sterols implicated in lowering cholesterol levels. They are relatively high in the amino acid arginine, a compound that relaxes blood vessels, helps to maintain flexible arteries and enhance blood flow.

Where to buy it: At the grocery store.

How much to eat: One 1 ounce serving of pistachios equals about 49 nuts. Consider having pistachio nuts as an afternoon snack three to four times weekly.

 Quick Tip 1: One serving of pistachios has as much potassium as half of a large banana. The next time you feel you need more potassium, reach for a handful of pistachios as an alternative.

 Quick Tip 2: Myth-Buster. When your mom told you to eat a banana (for the potassium) to relieve muscle cramps, she was right—sort of. Low potassium levels occasionally do cause muscle cramps, but more often low potassium is associated with muscle fatigue.

Salmon

Why: The omega-3 fats found in salmon are incredibly beneficial in protecting against cardiovascular disease. Omega-3s help prevent erratic heart rhythms, make blood less likely to clot inside arteries and improve the ratio of good cholesterol to bad cholesterol. Salmon is also a great source of protein, B vitamins, niacin and vitamin B12, L-carnitine and L-taurine—necessary nutrients for good heart function.

Where to buy it: At the grocery store. The preferred choice is fresh, wild salmon if available, but frozen or even canned wild salmon has incredible nutritional value.

How much to eat: Eating one 4-ounce portion three to four times a week is ideal.

Quick Tip: Eating as little as one serving a week of fish lowers the risk of ischemic ("is•skeem•ic") stroke (occurring when an artery to the brain is blocked).

Quick Fact 1: According to a Harvard study in 2004, eating baked or broiled salmon may reduce the risk of atrial fibrillation by 28%, the most common type of heart arrhythmia (particularly in the elderly). In a 12-year study of 4,815 people 65 years or older, eating canned tuna or other broiled or baked fish one to four times a week correlated with increased blood levels of omega-3 fatty acids. Eating broiled or baked fish five times a week lowered the risk even more-dropping atrial fibrillation risk by 31%.

Quick Fact 2: Whenever possible, choose wild rather than farm-raised salmon. Research published by the Environmental Working Group (July 30, 2003) indicates that farmed salmon poses a cancer risk because they carry high levels of carcinogenic chemicals called polychlorinated biphenyls (PCBs). PCBs have been banned in the US since 1979, but they persist in the environment and end up in animal fat. Farmed salmon from U.S. grocery stores contains 16 times the PCBs found in wild salmon.

Scallops

Why: Go ahead and indulge–scallops are a good source of vitamin B12, needed by the body to convert homocysteine, a chemical that damages blood vessel walls. High levels of homocysteine increases your risk for atherosclerosis, diabetic heart disease, heart attack and stroke. Scallops are also a great source of protein, omega-3s and magnesium–an important nutrient for relaxing blood vessels. Scallops also offer potassium which helps to maintain normal blood pressure levels.

Where to buy it: Either the fresh seafood or frozen section of your grocery store.

How much to eat: Four ounces of scallops contains 33.3% of the daily value for vitamin B12.

Quick Tip 1: Scallops are found in many waters throughout the world. The great scallop is abundant in the Mediterranean, whereas the sea and bay scallop are found concentrated in the Atlantic Ocean off North America.

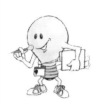

Quick Tip 2: Simple changes in your diet can reduce cholesterol consumption to 300 mg a day (the recommended daily amount). Seafood fits right in when trying to meet these dietary goals. Below are average amounts of cholesterol (from lowest to highest) for a 3 ½ ounce portion:

- Fish = 50–90 mg
- Mollusks (clams, oysters, scallops) = 40–110 mg
- Shellfish (crab, lobsters, shrimp) = 60–100 mg
- Squid and octopus = 122–250 mg

Sunflower Seeds

Why: Sunflower seeds are loaded with heart protective nutrients, providing protein, fiber, vitamin E, folic acid and many of the B vitamins, the minerals selenium, copper, phosphorous, iron, magnesium and zinc. All these nutrients keep your heart muscles running smoothly and your blood pressure levels down.

Where to buy it: At the grocery store; purchase unsalted.

How much to eat: Just one ¼ cup of sunflower seeds contains 18 IU of vitamin E, 127 mg of magnesium, 22 mcg of selenium, 82 mcg of folic acid. Sunflower seeds are an excellent choice for an afternoon snack or added to your favorite salad.

Quick Tip: Because sunflower seeds have a high fat content and therefore prone to rancidity, store them in an airtight container in the refrigerator or freezer. The cold temperature won't affect their flavor.

Water, Water, Water

Why: According to a 2002 study in the *American Journal of Epidemiology*, "Water, Other Fluids and Fatal Coronary Disease," people who drink five or more glasses of water a day (not tea, coffee, or even scotch and water) have a much lower risk of fatal coronary heart disease compared to those who drink less than two glasses per day. The study also shows that by drinking more water, people reduce their risk of dying from a heart attack by 50% or more.

Where to buy it: This incredible liquid is found right in your own home.

How much to drink: Drink at least ½ your body weight in ounces daily, i.e., 150 pounds divided in half = 75 pounds; next, convert that to ounces = 75 ounces/day. A medium sized bottle of water is approximately 25 ounces. So you should drink **three** of those each day.

 Quick Tip: Keep in mind that thirst is an indicator of dehydration; it is not an early warning sign. By the time you feel thirsty, you may already be dehydrated. Other symptoms of dehydration include: dizziness and lightheadedness, having a dry or sticky mouth and/or producing less and darker urine.

Nutrients for Heart Health

EFAs

Probably the most important nutrient for heart health, EFAs help to:

- Reduce inflammation throughout the body
- Keep blood from excessive clotting
- Maintain the fluidity of cell membranes
- Lower the amount of lipids (fats such as cholesterol and triglycerides) circulating in the bloodstream
- Decrease platelet aggregation
- Inhibit thickening of the arteries
- Increase the activity of nitric oxide in the endothelial cells, helping the arteries to relax and dilate

Co Q 10

An important nutrient for our heart health and blood vessels, CoQ10 lies at the heart of our cells' energy-producing process. In heart cells, this energy conversion process can be the difference between life and death. The CoQ10 antioxidants provide protection from oxygen damage in the heart muscle as well as other conditions including arrhythmia, angina, heart attack, mitral valve prolapse, high blood pressure, coronary artery disease, atherosclerosis, and congestive heart failure. It also revitalizes vitamin E in the body. (Rather than vitamin E being used up after it attaches to free radicals in the body, it is able to go out again and attach to another free radical.)

Magnesium

Magnesium performs hundreds of important jobs in the body, including energy production, the functioning of the heart, nerves, and muscles, bone health, the clotting of blood and regulating blood pressure. Magnesium is important for the nerves that initiate the heartbeat, preventing arrhythmias and keeping blood vessels healthy to prevent spasms of coronary arteries, causing angina.

Folic Acid

Folic acid assists in maintaining normal homocysteine levels (an amino acid in the blood). Among other things, homocysteine accelerates the oxidation of LDL ("Lousy") cholesterol that damages arteries.

Q*uick Tip*: What's Oxidation? It's a natural process and a by-product of the body's function. Think of it this way, your outside water pipes get some added rust on them from everyday wear and tear and environmental factors. If you live in an area where there is lots of salt air, more rust occurs than if you live in a desert community. This rusting is oxidation. In our body, we develop oxidation (rusting) similar to the outside pipes. The difference is we can feed our body with antioxidants (from many vegetables and fruits) to help fight this oxidation process, slowing down the rusting, or aging process.

Vitamin B12

B12 works along with folic acid and vitamin B6 to convert homocysteine into a harmless compound that the body can eliminate through urination.

Vitamin B6

In addition to helping to keep homocysteine levels in check, vitamin B6 helps promote healthy adrenal function and maintains proper potassium balance. Potassium helps support normal heart rhythms and regulates blood pressure levels.

Lycopene

Before cholesterol can be collected in the plaques that harden and narrow arteries, it must be oxidized by free radicals. Lycopene, with its powerful antioxidant activity, can prevent LDL cholesterol from being oxidized.

L-Carnitine

Studies suggest that people who take L-carnitine supplements soon after suffering a heart attack may be less likely to suffer a subsequent heart attack, die of heart disease, experience chest pain and abnormal heart rhythms or develop congestive heart failure. L-carnitine supplements create lower total cholesterol, triglycerides and an increase in HDL ("good") cholesterol. In addition, coronary artery disease sufferers using L-carnitine, along with standard medications, may be able to sustain physical activity for longer periods of time.

L-Taurine

L-taurine helps support proper heart function by normalizing potassium flow in and out of the heart muscle and aiding in free-radical elimination.

High Fiber Foods

A culmination of 10 studies, published in a February 2004 issue of the *Archives of Internal Medicine* showed that dietary fiber from cereals and fruits are associated with reduced risk of heart disease. Almost 100,000 men and more than 245,000 women studied showed that for every ten grams of daily fiber consumed from cereals and fruits, the risk of all coronary disease dropped 14% and risk of death from heart attack dropped 27%.

Fiber is present in all plants that are eaten for food including fruits, vegetables, grains and legumes. However, not all fiber is the same, and there are a number of ways to categorize it. One is by its source or origin. For example, fiber from grains is referred to as cereal fiber. Another way of categorizing fiber is by how easily it dissolves in water.

Soluble fiber partially dissolves in water while insoluble fiber does not. These differences are important when it comes to fiber's effect on your risk of developing certain diseases.

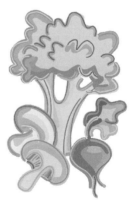

Soluble fiber in the intestines binds to bile from the liver. The bile is then carried out of the body as waste instead of being reabsorbed. In order for the body to make more bile, necessary for digestion, it must break down more cholesterol, removing it from the bloodstream.

Quick Tip: Soluble fiber significantly reduces blood cholesterol levels in several different ways. It:
(1) Decreases the absorption of dietary cholesterol.
(2) Increases the breakdown of blood cholesterol to produce more bile.
(3) Increases the removal of bile.
(4) Decreases the activity HMG Co-A reductase, a key enzyme involved in the production of cholesterol by the liver.

Antioxidants

We produce millions of free radicals every second. If free radicals aren't eliminated from the body they can cause cell mutations and aging. Antioxidants rid the body of free radicals–kind of like super heroes who seize the bad guys and then usher them out as waste.

Consuming more antioxidants provides the body with tools to neutralize harmful free radicals. It's estimated that there are more than 4,000 antioxidant compounds in foods and it's been found that obtaining antioxidants from foods is much more effective than getting them from isolated supplements. The most studied include vitamins C, E, beta-carotene and selenium. Foods scoring high in an antioxidant analysis called ORAC (Oxygen Radical Absorbance Capacity) protect cells and their components from damage. In recent studies eating plenty of high ORAC foods raised the antioxidant power of human blood 10 to 25 percent.

Good Cholesterol – Bad Cholesterol?
That is the Question!

So what is cholesterol? Found in every cell in the body, cholesterol is a type of lipid (fatty substance) that's soft and waxy. It forms cell membranes, sex and stress reaction hormones, and it also makes vitamin D. Cholesterol is produced in the liver or it can be obtained from eating animal products. Cholesterol and other fats need transportation to go from cell to cell. These carriers are called lipoproteins–low-density lipoprotein (LDL) and high-density lipoprotein (HDL). LDL is the major cholesterol carrier in the blood.

HDL is the collector; it travels throughout the body collecting the extra cholesterol not used by cells (for this reason, HDL is often referred to as the "healthy" or good cholesterol). The HDL takes its collected cholesterol to the liver where it's transformed and used again by the body. *Here's where you might begin to feel like you're in a maze...hang in there...*Next, the liver converts the collected cholesterol to bile and stores it in the gall bladder until it's needed in the intestines where it helps digest fats. *Still with me?* The important thing to remember: it's easy to get out of balance when we feed our body too much cholesterol from highly saturated fats. We get an overload of cholesterol in our blood and don't have enough of the HDL to carry it to the liver. Here's a visual to help explain:

Think of LDL as the trains that drop off cholesterol for the cells to use as needed. HDL are the buses that go around and pick up extra, unused cholesterol and transport them to the liver. If there aren't enough HDL buses to do the job (or they get overloaded), cholesterol sits and waits around for the next bus. While waiting, they cause trouble by building small "tents" on the artery walls, resulting in blockages. Eating foods with high HDL, and low LDL ensures no cholesterol camping happens in your arteries!

 ***Quick Tip:* Understanding your cholesterol numbers:** Think of LDL as the *Lousy* cholesterol and HDL as *Healthy* cholesterol. The recommended ratio is under five to one (LDL to HDL). Your doctor can give you your cholesterol levels with a simple blood test.

What does all of this cholesterol have to do with heart health? The higher the blood cholesterol level, the greater the risks for developing heart disease or having a heart attack. Heart disease is the number one killer of women and men in the United States. It's estimated that half million people die annually from heart disease and more than a million Americans have heart attacks each year.

——————— And the Beat Goes On... ———————

Blood Pressure

Everybody has, and needs, blood pressure. Without it, blood can't circulate through the body, and without circulating blood, vital organs can't get the oxygen and food that they need to work. For this reason, it's important to know about blood pressure and how to keep it within a healthy level.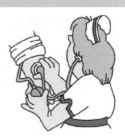

When the heart beats, it pumps blood through the arteries and creates pressure in them. This blood pressure results from two forces: (1) as blood pumps into the arteries and through the circulatory system, and (2) as the arteries resist the blood flow. A normal heart beats about 60 to 80 times per minute. Blood pressure rises with each heartbeat and falls when the heart relaxes between beats. Blood pressure can also change from minute to minute, affected by things like a change in posture, exercise, stress or sleeping. Normal ranges for an adult are somewhere around 120/80 mm Hg.

> **Quick Tip:**
> - The higher, systolic (or first) represents the pressure while the heart is beating.
> - The lower, diastolic (or second) number represents the pressure when the heart is resting between beats.

Certain nerve impulses cause your arteries to dilate (become larger) or contract (become smaller). If these vessels are wide open, blood flows easily. If they're narrow, it's harder for the blood to flow through them, and the pressure inside them increases. High blood pressure may result. When this happens, the heart is strained and blood vessels may become damaged. However, the heart, brain and kidneys can handle increased pressure for a long time. That's why you can live for years without any symptoms. And experiencing no symptoms doesn't mean there's no damage. Also, blood pressure is a function of arteries flexibility, the more flexible the arteries the lower the pressure. High blood pressure is a major risk factor for stroke, heart attack, heart failure and kidney failure.

If you find you have high blood pressure, you can do several things to reduce it:

- Reduce fat (particularly saturated fat) in your diet
- Eat less salt
- Change your lifestyle by losing weight and getting regular physical activity
- Quit smoking
- Keep alcohol consumption to 1 to 2 ounces daily

As you can see, it's easier and healthier to maintain a healthy blood pressure level with food and lifestyle, rather than relying on many medications.

The Heart of the Matter

Atherosclerosis

The name comes from the Greek words athero (meaning gruel or paste) and sclerosis (hardness). It's the term for fatty substances, cholesterol, cellular waste products, calcium and fibrin (a clotting material in the blood) that build up in the inner lining of an artery. This buildup is called plaque, a common disorder of the arteries. The vessel walls become thick and hardened and the vessel narrows. This lessens circulation (nutrients and oxygen) to organs and other areas normally supplied by the artery. This plaque (atheromas) is a major cause of heart disease, chest pain (angina pectoris) and heart attacks. Some hardening of arteries occurs normally as we age. Exactly how atherosclerosis begins or what causes it isn't entirely known. It's thought that atherosclerosis may even start in childhood and as a slow, progressive disease that goes undetected until later in life. Other scientists believe atherosclerosis starts because the innermost layer of the artery becomes damaged. This layer is called the endothelium. Three possible causes of damage to the arterial wall are:

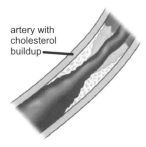

artery with cholesterol buildup

- Elevated levels of cholesterol and triglyceride in the blood
- High blood pressure
- Cigarette smoke or smoking cigarettes

Not all Fats are Created Equal

With all the bad press fat has gotten over the last couple of decades, most Americans have concluded that just limiting fats makes a diet healthy. This isn't true. Limiting saturated fats (meat and dairy) and avoiding transaturated fats is most important (see Trans Fats: The Ugly Truth on p.95). Oils, like olive oil and omega-3 fish oils, are good for both blood vessels and waistlines. First, let's take a look at the different types of fats.

Saturated fatty acids are found mainly in animal fats like dairy, cheese, butter, whole milk and fatty meats as well as in tropical oils like coconut oil, palm oil and palm kernel oils. These fatty acids are compact in structure, making them extremely stable even in high temperatures. The good news for saturated fatty acids is that cooking them at high temperatures does not alter their properties and is considered safe to consume in low quantities. **Saturated fats raise your blood cholesterol level more than anything else in your diet.** So, the best way to reduce your cholesterol level is to cut back on the amount of saturated fats that you eat.

Monounsaturated fatty acids (good fats) are usually liquid at room temperature and are relatively stable even when exposed to heat. The most common type of monounsaturated fatty acid found in food is called oleic acid. Monounsaturated fatty acids are found in olive oil, avocados, peanuts, almonds, pecans and cashews. **These are good fats and can be consumed in moderation but they all do yield high calories.**

Polyunsaturated fatty acids remain liquid even in the refrigerator, are highly unstable and go bad quite easily when exposed to heat and light. The most common polyunsaturated fatty acids found in our foods are omega-6 and omega-3 fatty acids. These fatty acids are considered to be essential fatty acids because the body cannot make them on its own. They must be obtained through diet. It's important to maintain a balance of omega-6 and omega-3 with an optimal ratio of 1:1. Maintain this healthy ratio by eating a well balanced diet of whole, relatively unprocessed foods, and vegetables, along with smaller amounts of fruits, legumes, nuts, seeds, whole grains and organic or wild animal products, including cold-water fish. Also consider using a high-quality cod liver oil as it contains an abundance of omega-3. **Polyunsaturated fatty acids play a primary role in development and proper functioning of the nervous system, inflammation and immunity. Consuming omega-3s in your daily diet is essential to good health.**

 Quick Tip: Adding omega-3s from fish oil supplements (in the dose of 2800 to 6000 mg) per day is ideal. Break this up between morning and evening. Two tablespoons of flax seed oil combined with a morning shake is also a good way of getting omega-3s, or add 3 to 4 tablespoons of freshly ground flax seed. Ground flax seed is also a good source of fiber.

Keep in mind that all fats and oils from animal and plant sources are made up of a combination of all three types of fatty acids. Eat high quality fats like fish oil, flax oil and seeds, almonds, walnuts, avocados and olive oils.

─────── News for Vegetarians ───────

Vegetarians and vegans have no direct sources of eicosapentaenoic acid (EPA) and docosahexaenoic acid (DHA) (long chain omega-3 fatty acids) in the diet. So they must convert alpha-linolenic acid to EPA and DHA in the body.

Scientific studies suggest that although the conversion to EPA and DHA is slow and incomplete (possibly only 10% of alpha-linolenic acid is converted), and although vegetarians tend to have lower blood levels of long chain omega-3 fatty acids, it is adequate to meet the needs of most people.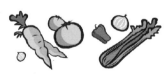

Making monounsaturated fats the principal fat in the diet helps get the omega-3s needed. Good sources of monounsaturated fats are olive oil (77% mono-fat) and/or canola oil (58% mono-fat). Avocados, olives, hazelnuts, pistachios, almonds, macadamia nuts, peanuts and pecans are also excellent sources of monounsaturated fats. These foods also provide valuable vitamins, minerals, phytochemicals and fiber. When used moderately, they make an excellent addition to the vegetarian diet.

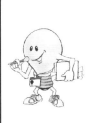

Quick Tip: The best source of alpha-linolenic acid is flaxseed oil (57% omega-3 and 17% omega-6 fatty acids). It works well as a salad dressing base or can be mixed with butter or a non-hydrogenated margarine for an omega-3-rich spread. Caution: The oil from flaxseed is highly unsaturated and easily damaged upon exposure to light, heat or air. It's found in the refrigerated section of natural food stores and is usually packaged in black plastic bottles or dark brown glass bottles to protect it from light. Refrigerate flaxseed oil for up to eight weeks after it's opened.

Trans Fats: The Ugly Truth

Trans fats are man-made or processed fats, made from liquid oil. When hydrogen is added to liquid vegetable oil and then pressurized, the result is a stiffer fat (like the fat found in a can of lard). Trans fats are also called hydrogenated fats or oils. Common names for trans fats include:

- Partially hydrogenated soybean oil
- Hydrogenated corn oil
- Hydrogenated soybean
- Hydrogenated cottonseed oil
- Hydrogenated palm kernel oil
- Hydrogenated coconut oil
- Hydrogenated vegetable oil shortening.

Food manufacturers started putting them in products because they allow for a longer shelf life, reduced cost, and improved flavor and texture. Crackers, for example, can stay on the shelf and remain crispy for years, in part, because of the hydrogenated fats in them (a typical French fry has about 40% trans fatty acids). Trans fats are found in just about everything: cookies, crackers, icing, potato chips, margarine, microwave popcorn, some cereals, waffles, fried foods, doughnuts, muffins, pastries, some candies, ice cream, cakes, refrigerated cookie dough, cheese, pretzel and cracker kits, cheese puffs, chocolate or yogurt-covered snacks, corn chips, pudding snacks, weight-loss snack bars, nacho cheese dips, pizza and pizza crusts, pot pies, refrigerated non-dairy creamers, some salad dressings, boxed onion soup and dip mixes, certain types of noodle and soup cups and the list goes on! In fact, it may be easier to mention the products that don't have trans fats...

Trans fats increase the blood's level of low density lipoprotein (LDL or "Lousy") cholesterol, while lowering levels of high density lipoprotein (HDL, "healthy") cholesterol. They do the same thing in our bodies that bacon grease does to kitchen drains. It can cause major clogging of arteries, Type-II diabetes and an increased risk of heart disease, among other serious health problems. Children who begin a steady diet of fast food and chips at age three or four can expect to get heart disease earlier than kids who are eating foods without trans fats. And although heart disease may not show up until around age 40, some research shows that kids as young as eight, nine and ten already have the high cholesterol and blood fats that clog arteries. It's important to start healthy eating habits early to help avoid heart attacks and strokes. If you haven't started yet, get busy!

Quick Facts: Because of the potentially serious health threat of trans fats, the U.S. Food and Drug Administration (FDA) required that beginning in 2006 any product containing trans fatty acids be labeled accordingly.

————— You Make My Heart Race ... —————

Exercising is as important for your heart as making the right choices in what you eat! Exercise makes your heart stronger by pumping more blood with each heartbeat, delivering more oxygen to your body. Exercise can also lower blood pressure, reduce your risk of heart disease and reduce levels of LDL ("Lousy") cholesterol. At the same time, exercise raises levels of HDL ("Healthy") cholesterol.

The good news is that taking a brisk walk for as little as 20 minutes a day will reduce the risk of cardiovascular disease.

Quick Facts: The Institute of Medicine, as reported in the *New England Journal of Medicine*, wrote that of 73,743 women, followed for a number of years, those who reported walking at least 2.5 hours a week (roughly 20 minutes a day) reduced their cardiovascular risk by 30%.

Exercise and Nitric Oxide

Reports also show exercise increases nitric oxide levels in the blood. Nitric oxide protects the artery lining, especially for those who are labeled "at risk" for heart disease. It's released by the endothelium—the lining of artery walls—and works to prevent red blood cells from sticking together and attaching to the vessel wall. Nitric oxide also works to control vascular tone, allowing the arteries to relax and stay clear.

Quick Tip: The drug Viagra was initially developed to help increase nitric oxide for cardiovascular health. With that success came the realization that the increased levels of nitric oxide and smooth muscle relaxation allowed extra blood flow to the penis. This led to an erection (much to their probable delight) and millions of dollars in product sales. Exercising daily not only helps reduce cardiovascular disease, but may be just as helpful in increasing sexual performance.

Exercise that conditions the heart and lungs	Exercise that helps condition the heart and lungs moderately
Aerobic Dancing	Basketball
Bicycling	Calisthenics
Cross-Country Skiing	Downhill Skiing
Hiking (uphill)	Field Hockey
Ice Hockey	Handball
Jogging	Racquetball
Jumping Rope	Soccer
Rowing	Squash
Running in Place	Tennis (singles)
Stair-climbing	Volleyball
Stationary Cycling	Walking Moderately
Swimming	
Walking Briskly	

Chapter 6

···

Superfoods for the Immune System

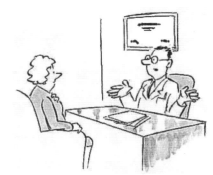

"ACCORDING TO ALL OUR TESTS, YOUR
IMMUNE SYSTEM IS OUT TO LUNCH"

When viruses, bacteria and allergies assault our bodies, we have a huge variety of responses available to combat them. Over-the-counter medications mainly deal with symptoms. When we're under the weather, staying in our pajamas, nesting in bed, enjoying the guilty pleasure of day time TV, and escaping from it all makes the experience nearly bearable. This "down time" is essential. The immune system needs quiet in order for it to do its job. Though you may need to think and work while you recuperate, the immune system would rather you didn't.

Many people have poor eating habits that cause nutritional imbalances and weaken the immune system. A weakened immune system resembles a rusty gate hanging on broken hinges. The wall may be stout but invaders can saunter in at will making us sick and miserable. If we're healthy, the gate slams shut and is secured with a big lock. Think of a good immune system as a strong wall, the interior accessible only through a massive, electrified gate and only nutritionally sound meals are allowed in!

There are Superfoods that give our immune system extra ammunition to fight off viruses, bacteria and toxins. Nutritionists and dieticians have long recommended quality nutrient intake to positively affect human immune factors. Important nutrient intake of vitamins A, Bs, C and E, zinc, iron, selenium plus powerful antioxidants, bioflavonoids and carotenoids all contribute to enhancing the immune system.

Quick Facts: Professors at Harvard University have published considerable evidence in the prestigious *New England Journal of Medicine* showing that 90% of all cancer is environmentally (the air we breathe, food, water, etc.) caused and therefore preventable. They cite how breast cancer has risen 500% in the last 20 years. This increase is thought to be related to diet. They highlight EFAs, selenium, vitamins A, C and E, along with fiber, as nutritionally proven cancer preventions.

Immune Bits

- ✓ A cold is a contagious viral disease which infects the soft lining (mucous membrane) of the nose. There are more than 200 different viruses that can result in a cold.
- ✓ Your body's resistance to contracting a cold is not affected by being wet or chilled. Catching a cold is not related to cold temperatures or bad weather, but rather is an actual virus caught by touching or breathing it in.
- ✓ The "Cold Season" lasts from September to March. Eighty percent of all annual colds are contracted during this time period; however, summer colds are not uncommon
- ✓ The U.S. Centers for Disease Control and Prevention (CDC) estimates that 35 to 50 million Americans come down with the flu during each flu season, which typically lasts from November to March.
- ✓ The American Academy of Allergy, Asthma and Immunology (AAAAI) estimates that 40 to 50 million people in the United States suffer from allergies.
- ✓ Many plants carry pollens that can trigger allergies, but ragweed is the most common. In fact, 75% of people with seasonal allergies are allergic to ragweed, according to the Asthma and Allergy Foundation of America (AAFA).
- ✓ An autoimmune disease can happen when our own immune system gets confused and starts attacking our own joints, muscles, blood vessels or kidneys.

Superfoods for Immune System

Astragalus *(as•TRAG•a•lus)*

Why: This incredible herb is well known as an immune stimulant. Scientific studies have documented a strong immune-enhancing effect of the herb thought to be associated with its polysaccharide contents.

Where to buy it: The health food store or you can buy it from www.mountainrose.com in a sliced form.

How much to take/eat: As a tonic, take 60 mg daily. For a more therapeutic dose, take 500 mg daily. Also add astragalus to soups, as cooking does not affect its valuable properties.

Quick Facts: Perhaps the best evidence to date for the powerful immunostimulant effects of astragalus comes from the University of Texas Medical Center in Houston. Scientists there tested damaged immune system cells from cancer patients and compared them against blood cells from normal human subjects. Astragalus extracts were able to completely restore the function of cancer patients' immune cells. In some cases, the compromised cells were stimulated to greater activity than those from normal human subjects. The study concluded, "A complete immune restoration can be achieved by using a fractionated extract of Astragalus membranaceus, a traditional Chinese medicinal herb found to possess immune restorative activity in vitro."

Barley Grass

Why: Barley grass is thought to stimulate the production of Interleukin 2 (Interleukin 2 enables the body's T-cells to kill cancer cells, T-cells don't normally have this ability). Barley grass has one of the highest natural levels of enzyme SOD (superoxide dismutase), a powerful antioxidant that protects the cells against toxic free radicals. It contains chlorophyll, a natural detoxifier that rids the intestines of stored toxins, and barley grass is rich in other immune nutrients like iron, all the essential amino acids, flavonoids, the B vitamins and vitamin C.

Where to buy it: At health food stores and some progressive grocery stores. A good Superfood drink is another excellent way to get your daily dose of barley grass.

How much to take/eat: Because all products are different, it's best to follow the recommended dose on the product's package.

> *Quick Facts:* A biologist named Yasuo Hotta from the University of California, La Jolla found barley grass contains a substance called P4D1. This substance not only has strong anti-inflammatory action, but also was shown to repair the DNA in the cells of the body. This aided in the prevention of abnormal growths, aging and cell death. He reported at a Japan Pharmacy Science Association meeting that P4D1 suppresses or cures pancreatitis, stomachitis, inflammation of the oral cavity, dermatitis and also lacerations of the stomach and duodenum. He found that barley grass juice is much stronger than steroid drugs, but has fewer, if any, side effects.

Broccoli

Why: Broccoli contains all the necessary nutrients, vitamins A, Bs, C and E, omega-3s, zinc and iron and some protein to boost the immune system. Research has shown the cruciferous vegetables, like broccoli, contain the phytochemicals, sulforaphane and the indoles, all providing valuable anti-cancer effects.

Where to buy it: The fresh produce section of the grocery store.

How much to eat: A ½ cup a day, cooked or raw, gives you great immune protection. Some of the health-supporting compounds in broccoli can be increased by slicing or chewing, as both slicing and chewing help activate its enzymes.

> *Quick Facts:* When researchers at Johns Hopkins studied the effect of sulphoraphane on tumor formation in lab animals, those animals given sulforaphane had fewer tumors. And the tumors they did develop grew more slowly and were smaller in size.

> *Quick Facts:* A study published December 2003 in the cancer journal *Oncology Report,* demonstrated that sulforaphane is a potent inducer of Phase 2 liver detoxification enzymes. It also induces cell death of abnormal cells in both leukemia and melanoma cells.

Carrots

Why: Carrots are a rich source of carotenoids. One cup provides over 16,000 IU (international units). High carotenoid intake has been linked with a 20% decrease in postmenopausal breast cancer and up to a 50% decrease in the incidence of cancers of the bladder, cervix, prostate, colon, larynx and esophagus. Carrots' protective effects are the result of a team effort among several substances abundant in carrots, including alpha-carotene-another, less publicized carotenoid. Carrots also contain significant levels of lutein and zeaxanthin found to inhibit development of colon cancer.

Where to buy it: In the fresh produce section of the grocery store.

How much to eat: Eating one carrot per day serves as one of your 8 to 10 daily recommended fruits and vegetables.

> ***Quick Facts:*** A research study reported in the 2000 *American Journal of Clinical Nutrition* examined the dietary habits of 1,993 patients with colon cancer and 2,410 cancer-free participants. Researchers weighed information gathered against cancer occurrence, stage and prognosis for all study participants and found that when a daily diet contained ample sources of lutein, men and women are 17% less likely to develop colon cancer. Zeaxanthin was also shown to be protective against colon cancer. Cancer patients whose colon cancer developed before they had reached the age of 67, or whose tumors occurred further up the colon, obtained the most significant benefits from lutein.

Chlorella *(chlo•rel•la)*

Why: Research has shown that Chlorella is a powerful immunostimulant, a strong detoxifier and has wound-healing properties. Chlorella contains more chlorophyll per gram than any other plant.

Where to buy it: In the health food stores, usually found in tablet, capsule or powdered form. It's also often one of the main ingredients found in Superfood drinks.

How much to eat: Follow the recommended product packaging amounts.

> ***Quick Tip:*** Chlorophyll is one of the greatest food substances for cleansing the bowel and other elimination systems, such as the liver and the blood.

> ***Quick Facts:*** A research study in 1998 done in Japan found that chlorella enhances the production of T-cell activation in the lymphoid organs, helping to prevent cancer cells from metastasis (duplicating and spreading). It also suggested that pre-surgical treatment with chlorella might prevent metastasis or tumor progression.

Mushrooms

Why: Shiitake mushrooms contain an active compound called lentinan, which supports the immune system and strengthens its ability to fight infection and disease. Lentinan has been shown to be as effective as prescription drugs against viruses. Another important compound–found in certain types of mushrooms like portabellas, crimninis, oyster and maitake–is L-ergothioneine, a powerful antioxidant found to protect liver function.

Where to buy it: At the grocery store; many shiitake mushrooms are dried and found in packages in the international food section. Dried shiitake contains the same great benefits.

How much to eat: Eat a ¼ cup serving three to four times a week.

Quick Facts: In testing mushrooms consumed in the U.S., the research presented at the American Chemical Society meeting in Washington, D.C., on August 31, 2005, found that shiitake, oyster, king oyster and maitake contain the highest amounts of L-ergothioneine, with up to 13 mg in a 3-ounce serving. This equals 40 times as much as is found in wheat germ. Of the most commonly consumed mushrooms, portabellas and criminis have the most L-ergothioneine, followed by white buttons. White buttons, the most popular of all mushrooms consumed in the U.S., contain up to five mg per 3-ounce serving12 times as much as wheat germ and four times more than chicken liver. And more good news, L-ergothioneine is not destroyed during cooking.

Fermented Foods

Why: Some fermented foods help the body make beneficial bacterium (probiotics). Probiotic's research has shown that adding "friendly" bacteria to the diet will improve the health of gut microflora and help protect both the lining of the intestinal tract and the immune system. Research has established that probiotics improve the body's ability to resist intestinal infection and improve digestion, help in absorption of nutrients and is important in the manufacturing of B vitamins and K vitamins. Plus, this good bacterium is essential in defending our body from viral attacks.

- **Kefir** is a fermented milk product which contains a unique mixture of several live microorganisms. It has all nutrients required by the body: proteins, minerals and vitamins and is highly digestible. Because of its acidity and enzymes, it stimulates digestion of other foods.

- o *Where to buy it:* Look for "Lifeway" brand found in Whole Foods Markets and other specialty health food markets.
- **Kimchi (kimchee)** is a condiment found in Korean cooking. Kimchi is a fermented combination of different foods mainly garlic, salt, chili, cabbage and rice vinegar. It's a highly nutritious, fermented food with a unique flavor and taste. Kimchi ingredients (like red pepper, garlic, ginger, green onion, etc.) facilitate the secretion of digestive enzymes and restrain the activation of poisonous bacteria. It also works to clean out your system by nourishing the lactobacteria and bifidobacteria so they can thrive and outnumber the "unfriendly bacteria" that live in the intestines.
  - o *Where to buy it:* You can find Kimchi at many grocery stores in the delicatessen area.
- **Yogurt** *Stonyfield* Yogurt contains six active cultures, providing a wide array of beneficial bacteria. Yogurt contains transient beneficial bacteria that keep the digestive system clean and provide food for the friendly bacteria that reside there. When purchasing yogurt look for the words that say it has *live acidophilus*, otherwise you're not getting the benefits of probiotics.
  - o *Where to buy it:* You can find *Stonyfield* yogurt at many specialty grocery stores in the delicatessen area.

How much to eat: Alternate between all of these probiotic foods (four to five servings) during the week in servings of a ½ to 1 cup each.

Prebiotic Foods

Why: The word prebiotic is generally defined as consisting of nondigestible food fibers which stimulate the growth and activity of certain bacteria in the intestine. The following foods are excellent sources of inulin, essential for prebiotics benefits:

- **Jerusalem Artichokes.** Also known as sunchokes, Jerusalem artichokes feed the healthy bacteria (lactobacilli) in the intestinal tract. They're also a great source of iron, potassium and B1 vitamin. Jerusalem artichokes have a high amount of inulin (a carbohydrate not used for energy production), which actually assists in blood sugar control. The root looks similar to ginger root, with light brown skin which may be tinged with yellow. It's very tasty added to salads.

- o *Where to buy it:* Some grocery stores and many specialty markets carry this delicious root in the produce section.

- **Chicory.** Also known as endive or radicchio, chicory is high in inulin which feeds the healthy bacteria in the intestines.

- o *Where to buy it:* It can be found in the fresh produce section of grocery stores. Add this inulin powerhouse to your salad mixture.

- **Burdock Root.** Also known as gobo, burdock root is also very high in inulin. Fresh burdock roots can destroy certain bacteria and fungi making it a good tonic on the fight against infection. It's also a very good source of potassium and a moderate source of iron.

- o *Where to buy it:* In the fresh produce section of Asian markets.

Quick Recipe
Hiroko's Kimpira Gobo

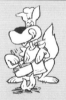

- 2 cups prepared burdock
- 2 cups prepared carrots
- 1 Tbsp vegetable oil
- 1 tsp sesame oil
- 2 Tbsp sesame seeds
- 1 Tbsp soy sauce

Prepare the burdock and carrots in the same way; wash and scrape the outer skin (don't peel), then cut into matchstick-size pieces.

After cutting burdock, throw the pieces into a bowl of cold water to prevent them from browning (browning occurs when burdock comes in contact with air).

In a large skillet or wok, heat the vegetable oil and sesame oil together. When hot, sprinkle in the sesame seeds and cook, stirring for about a minute.

Drain the burdock and carrots, placing them in the pan. Cook and stir over medium-high heat for about five to seven minutes.

Add soy sauce and continue stir-frying for about ten minutes. The burdock will change color from milky white to shiny gray/brown. The finished product is crisp, crunchy and delicious.

Quick Tip 1: After simmering the burdock root in water, the water makes a very useful remedy as well as the vegetable. Ingested together, they aid digestion and remove toxins from the body. Gargling with the simmered water is good for mouth ulcers, and when applied directly, burdock root juice counteracts insect bites and stinging nettles.

Quick Tip 2: Gobo (burdock root) has a tendency to taste bitter; soaking them in rice vinegar water will take the bitter edge off. Choose the straightest roots you can find, without cracks in the skin. Avoid hairy roots, as these are old.

Quick Facts: There is mounting scientific evidence that the symbiotic relationship between prebiotics and probiotics significantly contributes to health by having anticarcinogenic and antimicrobial benefits. Plus, they boost the immune system, help improve mineral absorption, rid the gut of harmful bacteria, help prevent constipation and diarrhea and help stabilize blood glucose levels.

Red Raspberries

Why: Clinical research indicates that red raspberries are the highest known source of the antioxidant, ellagic acid, which stimulates the production of glutathione (an antioxidant that protects cells from toxins such as free radicals). Ellagic acid inhibits the ability of other chemicals to cause mutations in bacteria and prevents binding of carcinogens to DNA, reducing incidence of cancer in human cells. 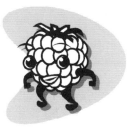 Raspberries are filled with nutrients that benefit the immune system including B and C vitamins. Red raspberries contain a powerful flavonoid, anthocyanins, a known antimicrobial that prevents overgrowth of certain bacteria and fungi in the body.

Where to buy it: At the grocery store.

How much to eat: A ½ cup, eaten four to five times a week counts as one of the 8 to 10 daily servings of vegetables and fruits.

Quick Tip: Fresh raspberries are very fragile, lasting only one to two days in the refrigerator. You can also buy them frozen. They're a wonderful addition to a nutrient shake.

Spirulina

Why: A nutrient-dense food with beneficial phytochemicals, researchers found that spirulina produces an immunostimulating effect by enhancing our resistance to infection by stimulating the production of antibodies, cytokines, macrophages, T and B cells. It's also been found to protect the liver, act as an anti-inflammatory and antioxidant. Spirulina has significant amounts of protein, essential amino acids, essential fatty acids, chlorophyll, carotenoids including beta-carotene, vitamins, minerals, unique pigments and polysaccharides. Spirulina also has probiotic compounds that enhance health through preserving resident intestinal microflora, especially lactic acid bacilli and bifidobacteria.

Where to buy it: At health food stores and sometimes drug stores. Spirulina is also found in Superfood drinks, tablets, capsules or powder form.

How much to eat: 500 mg to 2000 mg as a tonic (immune protector) is recommended.

Spinach

Why: Researchers have identified at least 13 different flavonoid compounds in spinach that function as antioxidants and anti-cancer agents. Spinach extracts have been shown to slow down cell division in stomach cancer cells (gastric adenocarcinomas), and in studies on mice, to reduce skin cancers (skin papillomas). A study on adult women living in New England in the late 1980s also showed the intake of spinach to be inversely related to incidence of breast cancer.

Where to buy it: In the fresh produce section or frozen food area of you grocery store.

How much to eat: A 1 cup serving, five to eight times a week.

 Quick Tip: In chemical pesticide testing of vegetables and fruits, spinach comes out rather high in pesticides. Whenever possible, purchase organic spinach.

Tomato, Cooked

Why: The carotenoid, lycopene, found in cooked tomato, has been extensively studied for its antioxidant and cancer-preventing properties. Lycopene helps protect cells and other structures in the body from oxygen damage and has been linked in human research to the protection of DNA (our genetic material) inside of white blood cells. Lycopene has been shown to help protect not only against prostate cancer, but breast, pancreatic and intestinal–especially when consumed with fat-rich foods, such as avocado, olive oil or nuts. This is because carotenoids are fat-soluble, meaning they are absorbed into the body along with fats. Tomatoes are also an excellent source of vitamin C, vitamin A and folic acid.

Where to buy it: At the grocery store in the canned food section.

How much to eat: A Harvard's Health Professionals Follow-up Study found that men who ate tomato sauce as little as once per week had a 23% lower prostate cancer risk than those who never ate it. Those men eating tomato-based products ten or more times per week were up to 35% less likely to develop prostate cancer. The study's lead author, Dr. Edward Giovannucci, believes that lycopene may be the key ingredient that causes this risk reduction.

Quick Tip: Cooked tomatoes found in ketchup, tomato sauce, sun dried tomatoes in olive oil are the best source of lycopene. Organic ketchup delivers three times as much of the cancer-fighting carotenoid, lycopene, as non-organic brands.

Turmeric

Why: The yellow or orange pigment of turmeric, called curcumin, is the primary pharmacological agent in turmeric. Epidemiological studies have linked the frequent use of turmeric to lower rates of breast, prostate, lung and colon cancer.

Quick Tip: In a laboratory study of human, non-Hodgkin's lymphoma cells published in the September 2005 issue of *Biochemical Pharmacology,* University of Texas researchers showed that curcumin is a powerful anti-inflammatory agent. This is significant in that inflammation is thought to contribute to cancer cell mutation.

Where to buy it: At the grocery store or Indian market.

How much to eat: ¼ to ½ teaspoon of the powder in a tea two to three times daily between meals. To make the tea, place ½ teaspoon of powder to 1 cup of boiling water, infuse for five minutes, strain and drink. You can add ginger or cardamom to add flavor.

Quick Tip: Turmeric can also be taken in capsules. Take 250-500 mg three times daily. Combining turmeric with bromelain enhances its absorption.

Quick Facts: Research has shown that combining turmeric's cancer-fighting agents with cruciferous vegetables (including cauliflower, cabbage, broccoli, Brussels sprouts, kale, kohlrabi and turnips) is a very effective therapy to inhibit the spread of established prostate cancer and also to help prevent it.

Myth: A bowl of chicken soup is a popular home remedy as an effective treatment for the flu or colds.

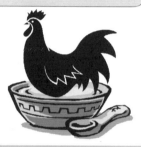

Fact: Although hot liquids can soothe a scratchy throat or cough, chicken soup has no special power to cure the flu or a cold.

Water

Why: No matter what the specific health or fitness goal, one cannot achieve the maximum benefit from any health program without drinking water in the proper amount. All experts agree, that next to the air we breathe, water is the most important thing we will ever put in our bodies. Isn't it surprising that so much time and money is being spent on supplements, organic foods and natural remedies (some of which are very subtle and delicate) but little attention is given to the quality and effect of the water with which those items are taken?

Where to buy it: At the grocery store. Drinking most any type of water is good, including tap water.

How much to drink: Drinking a one quart bottle of mineral water daily will provide important nutrients your body needs to maintain a healthy immune system.

Quick Facts: Dr. Batmanghelidj in his report "Medical Report: A New Medical Discovery" states, "Every function inside the body is regulated by and depends on water. Water must be available to carry vital elements, oxygen, hormones and chemical messengers to all parts of the body. Without sufficient water to wet all parts equally, some more remote parts of the body will not receive the vital elements that water supplies."

110

———— Nutrients for the Immune System ————

Vitamin C

Vitamin C has more research about its immune-boosting effects than perhaps any other nutrient. It increases the production of infection-fighting white blood cells and antibodies and increases levels of interferon (the antibody that coats cell surfaces preventing the entry of viruses). It's been found that as little as 200 mg a day (from food) boosts your immune system.

B Vitamins

Vitamin B5 (pantothenic acid) promotes the production and release of antibodies from B-cells (B cells react against invading bacteria and viruses.) Folic acid and vitamin B6 deficiency can lead to a decrease in T-cells. Deficiencies in vitamins B1(thiamin) and B2 (riboflavin) may impair normal antibody response, and low vitamin B12 appears to inhibit phagocytic cells (the white blood cells that eat up bacteria) and possibly T-cell function.

Vitamin E

Vitamin E stimulates the production of natural killer cells, which destroy germs and cancer cells. Vitamin E enhances the production of B-cells–the immune cells that produce antibodies to destroy bacteria.

Quick Facts: The immune system declines with aging, contributing to increased infections. Until now, few nutritional interventions have boosted older people's immune response. Reported in the *Journal of the American Medical Association* (vol. 277, pp. 1380-1386), a study of 80 volunteers took either 60, 200 or 800 mg of vitamin E-or a look-alike placebo–each day for 4½ months. They were then given a standard test, called DTH that measures the body's reaction to seven antigens injected into the skin. The DTH test indicates how well immune-system cells called T cells "remember" antigens they have seen before and how to respond to them. Compared with the placebo group, the group getting 200 mg daily–equivalent to 200 International Units–had a 65% increase in DTH response. Those taking 800 mg had a 49% increase, showing that more is *not* necessarily better.

Carotenoids

Beta carotene increases the number of infection-fighting cells, natural killer cells and helper T-cells, and is a powerful antioxidant. It protects against cancer by stimulating the immune cells called macrophages which kill cancer cells. Beta carotene is the most familiar carotenoid. *Researchers believe that it is not just beta carotene that produces all these good effects, but all the carotenoids working together.* This is why obtaining carotenoids from food is more cancer-protective than taking beta carotene supplements.

- The body converts beta carotene to vitamin A, which itself has anti-cancer properties and immune-boosting functions. It's highly unlikely that a person could take in too much beta carotene to produce a toxic amount of vitamin A because when the body has enough vitamin A, it stops producing it.

Bioflavonoids

Bioflavonoids are a group of phytonutrients found in brightly-colored fruits and vegetables that aid the immune system by protecting the cells of the body against environmental pollutants.

Iron

Low iron can increase the risk of infection and disease as our body does not work as efficiently without it.

Zinc

This indispensable mineral increases the production of white blood cells, helping them fight infection more aggressively. It also increases killer cells that fight against cancer. A word of caution: too much zinc in the form of supplements (more than 75 milligrams a day) can inhibit immune function. It's safest to stick to getting zinc from your diet, aiming for 15 to 25 milligrams a day.

Selenium

This mineral increases natural killer cells and mobilizes cancer-fighting cells.

Omega-3 Fatty Acids

They act as immune boosters by increasing the activity of phagocytes (the white blood cells that eat up bacteria).

Quick Facts: A study found that children taking ½ teaspoon of flax oil per day experienced fewer and less severe respiratory infections and had fewer days absent from school.

Protein

Protein is composed of the 20 amino acids the body needs for growth and repair. The amino acids, glutamine and arginine stimulate the immune system. Interestingly, it is not just deficiency of these amino acids that can compromise the immune system but imbalances in the ratios among amino acids also affect the immune response.

Quick Facts: Research studies have shown that a deficiency of high-quality protein can result in depletion of immune cells, the inability to make antibodies and other immune-related problems. In addition, animal studies have shown that the immune system can be significantly compromised with even a 25% reduction in adequate protein intake.

——— Immune Defense: The Constant Battle ———

The immune system is always on stand-by, ready to guard against invaders such as viruses, bacteria, infections, cuts, bug bites and toxins in the body. Poor eating habits, creating nutritional imbalances, are a major contributor to a weakened immune system.

 Quick Tip: When a mosquito bites, you get a red, itchy bump. That is a visible sign of the immune system at work.

Battle Stations! Germs are at the Gate!

The most obvious part of the immune system is your **skin**. It acts as a primary boundary between germs and the body, secreting antibacterial substances on its own. Our skin's pH is very acidic with an acid mantle of 4.5, which destroys many invading germs and stops mold from growing on us.

When you get a cut, all sorts of bacteria and viruses enter the body through the break in the skin. The immune system responds eliminating the invaders while the skin heals itself and seals the puncture. In rare cases, the immune system misses something and the cut gets infected. It gets inflamed and will often fill with pus. Inflammation and pus are both side effects of the immune system doing its job.

Your **nose, mouth and eyes** are the most common entry points for germs. Tears and mucus contain an enzyme (lysozyme) that breaks down the cell wall of many invading bacteria. Saliva in the mouth is also anti-bacterial. The nasal passage and lungs are coated in mucus. Many germs not killed immediately are trapped in the mucus and soon swallowed where the stomach acid takes care of them. Any bacteria or virus that wants to gain entry to the body must first make it past these many defenses.

✓ Each day you inhale thousands of germs (bacteria and viruses) floating in the air. Your immune system typically deals with all of them easily. Occasionally a germ slips past the immune system and you catch a cold, get the flu or worse. A cold or flu is a visible sign that your immune system failed to stop the germ. Recovery is a proof that your immune system was able to eliminate the invader. If your immune system were inactive, you would never get over a cold, or any other ailment.

✓ Each day you also eat hundreds of germs. Most of these die in the saliva or the acid of the stomach. Occasionally, however, one gets through and causes food poisoning. There are normally evident effects of this breach of the immune system: vomiting and diarrhea.

Once inside the body, the immune system deals with a germ at a different level. The major components of the immune system are:

✓ **Thymus.** Located in the chest, between your breast bone and your heart, the thymus is responsible for producing T-cells (white blood cells that attack viruses). As we age, the thymus becomes much smaller, seemingly much less important in adults. As an adult, the thymus can be removed and other parts of the immune system will handle the immune-fighting load.

> *Quick Tip*: Without a thymus, a baby's immune system collapses. In fact, the thymus of a newborn baby is the same size as the baby's heart!

✓ **Spleen.** While it's on the lookout for foreign cells, the spleen filters the blood of old red blood cells in need of replacement. When an invader is detected in the blood stream, the spleen, along with the lymph nodes, jump in to action and produce an army of defender cells–*blue print specific*–for that invader. These cells are released into the blood stream like homing missiles to attack and kill the invading germ.

✓ **Lymph system.** The lymph is often thought of as our second circulatory system, or our human garbage system. Its purpose is to fight infectious diseases. Any random bacteria that enter the body find their way into the lymph system. The lymph system drains and filters fluids as it detects and removes bacteria. Lymph fluid circulates through the system, coming from the blood and returning to the blood. In this way, the lymphatic fluid not only nourishes vital organs but also removes harmful substances from the body. There are over six hundred lymph nodes along our blood vessels throughout our body. They're bean shaped and are from ⅟₂₅ to 1 inch long.

 Quick Tip: Lymph flows slowly upward through the body to the top of the chest at a rate approximating 3 quarts per day.

✓ **Bone marrow.** Our bone marrow produces new blood cells, both red and white.

✓ **White blood cells.** These cells are actually a whole collection of different cells that work together to destroy bacteria and viruses in our body.

✓ **Antibodies.** Antibodies are produced by white blood cells. They respond to specific antigens (bacteria, virus or toxins) by binding to the cell wall, stopping the antigens' movement. Sometimes they call out for reinforcements to rid the body of the antigens.

✓ **Complement system.** Made up of antibodies, the complement system contains millions of different antibodies, each sensitive to a specific antigen. Manufactured in the liver, the complement proteins are activated by and "complement" the antibodies–hence its name.

✓ **Hormones.** There are several hormones generated by components of the immune system, known generally as lymphokines. They attract macrophages (our immune system's defense) to an affected site rendering the invaders harmless.

 Quick Tip:
Myth: "Feed a cold and starve a fever (flu)."
Fact: You need more fluids than usual when you have the flu or a cold. Drink plenty of water and juice, eat enough food to satisfy your appetite and drink hot fluids to ease your cough and sore throat.

115

A Confused Immune System

There are many human ailments caused by the immune system working in unexpected or incorrect ways. For example, some people have allergies. Allergies are really just the immune system overreacting to certain stimuli, where other people's immune system wouldn't react at all. Some people have rheumatoid arthritis, caused by the immune system acting inappropriately in the joints. In many different diseases, the cause is an immune system error.

The immune system can also be an obstacle because it prevents us from doing things that might be beneficial. For example, the immune system often attempts to reject transplanted organs.

Quick Facts: An autoimmune disorder is a disorder of the body's immune system in which the immune system mistakenly attacks and destroys body tissue that it believes to be foreign. Insulin-dependent diabetes is an autoimmune disease because the immune system attacks and destroys the insulin-producing beta cells. Multiple sclerosis is believed to be an autoimmune disease, along with systemic lupus, rheumatoid arthritis and scleroderma.

Quick Facts: Food allergies occur in roughly 1 to 2% of adults and 3 to 8% of children, according to the AAFA. About 90% of all food allergies have been traced to the following foods:

- Cow's milk
- Eggs
- Peanuts
- Tree nuts (e.g., almonds, walnuts)
- Wheat
- Soybeans
- Fish
- Shellfish

 Quick Tip: Many people confuse food allergy with food intolerance–a much more common condition and not as severe as an allergy. Food intolerance allows the individual to eat small portions of a food without experiencing symptoms. With a food allergy, even a very small portion causes an allergic reaction.

More Immune Ammunition

Exercise

Exercise has the capacity to protect and even enhance the immune response. Experimental studies have shown that a regular exercise program of brisk walking can bolster many defenses of the immune system, including the antibody response and the natural killer (T cell) response. Twenty to 30 minutes of brisk walking/five days per week is ideal for maintaining a healthy immune response. Exercise contributes to the pumping of lymph fluid in the body; muscles squeeze forcing waste and toxins out of the body.

Researchers are beginning to look at the effects moderate exercise has on the immune systems of cancer patients in the midst of their treatment. In one small study, researchers found that moderate exercise (three or more times a week) increased the immune cell counts of women undergoing breast cancer treatment back to normal levels, and also improved the women's mood and ability to deal with their emotional changes during this time.

Stress and Immunity

The final component for fine-tuning your immune system is to reduce the stress in your life. Altered mood states such as depression, anxiety and panic are harmful to the body in many ways. There are many techniques you can use to reduce stress and anxiety in your life. Guided imagery involves focusing on mental images, such as a serene setting. You can also try yoga or tai chi, which combine both mental and physical exercise, and can help heal the mind and the body. Other simple techniques include breathing exercises or taking a walk, appreciating the beauty of the world around you.

Laughter

Studies have shown that laughing lowers blood pressure, reduces stress hormones, increases muscle flexion, and boosts immune function by raising levels of infection-fighting T-cells which produce disease-destroying antibodies. Laughter also triggers the release of endorphins, the body's natural painkillers, producing a general sense of well-being.

To incorporate more laughter in your life, go back to Chapter Two and re-read "Laughter Fake it. Your Brain Won't Know the Difference!"

Chapter 7

. . . .

Superfoods for Weight Management and Metabolism

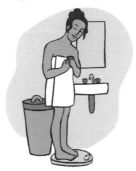

Planning proper exercise and good nutrition can seem daunting. Giving up our precious free time to jog, swim, do yoga or lift weights...and then...after all that, prepare a nutritious meal, discourages many of us before we even start. The reality, though, is quite different. The positive habits of eating right, managing weight and maintaining proper metabolism can simply *replace* those of lounging and overeating. Anticipating a brisk walk followed by a crisp salad with nuts and berries takes the same amount of brain power as heading for the couch to watch TV with a bag of chips. Did those chips really used to be potatoes? Not convinced yet? How about the way you'll feel after exercise and a nutritious meal as opposed to how you'll drag your semi-comatose self to bed after zoning out and binging? Need more incentive? What about the valuable time you'll save **not** sitting in the doctor's waiting room reading seven-month-old magazines? It takes practice, but replacing bad habits with better ones has many rewards. A lighter, leaner body is just one.

Weight: A Heavy Subject

✓ You're not alone in the battle against the bulge. More than ½ of all Americans start a weight reduction diet and nearly 50 million Americans are on a diet at any given time.

✓ A market research firm tracked diet programs and products and found that in 2004, $46.3 billion dollars were spent on the weight loss market. They went on to forecast that in 2008, $61 billion dollars will be spent annually on diets and weight loss products.

✓ About 80% of those on a weight loss program spend about three hours per week exercising. Walking is the exercise of choice.

119

- ✓ You burn about the same number of calories doing six sessions of an activity for five minutes OR doing one session for 30 minutes.
- ✓ New research findings suggest that controlling portion sizes may be the most effective thing a person can do to lose weight and keep it off. (Although increasing exercise is important, and does help people to lose weight, researchers found that for many obese individuals it was easier to reduce portion size than to increase physical activity.)
- ✓ Considered the first of its kind, a large, community-based study assessed the long-term risk of becoming overweight or obese. It found over a 30 year-period that nine out of ten men in the study (and seven out of ten women) were overweight or became overweight.
- ✓ Currently, one in six children/adolescents (17%) is significantly overweight.
- ✓ Reported in the *American Journal of Clinical Nutrition* (Feb. 2006), the increase in **excess** weight over the last four years was most pronounced in children and men. There was no significant change in obesity rates for women during this same period–surprising, isn't it?!

Quick Facts: A study of 7,194 men and women, ages 41 and older, were studied to see what foods were linked to weight gain. After 28 months of follow-up, here is what they found: The best predictor of weight gain was the intake of soda pop. People drinking the most soda were 60% more likely to gain a significant amount of weight during the study compared to those who seldom drank soda. Other foods positively linked to weight gain were hamburgers, pizza, sausage, red meat, and sweetened fruit juices. This shouldn't come as a surprise, but it certainly explains why Americans are gaining excess weight–these are among Americans' most favorite foods.

Superfoods for Weight Management and Metabolism

Adzuki Beans *(a•zu•ki)*

Why: Like most beans, Adzuki beans are rich in the best sort of fiber–soluble fiber–which helps to eliminate cholesterol (fats) from the body. They supply high-quality protein with less calories and fat, providing a healthy alternative to meat or other animal protein!

They're a good source of magnesium, potassium, iron, zinc, copper, manganese and vitamin B3, providing you with nutrients for energy.

Where to buy it: At the grocery store, in the dried foods section.

How much to eat: Eat 1 cup cooked beans, four to five times per week. Each cup provides 294 calories, 18 grams of protein, 56 grams of good carbs and no fat.

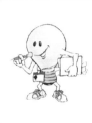
Quick Tip: Adzuki beans are easy to digest and have a distinctive flavor, tasting less "beany" than many other beans. The preferred cooking method is to soak them in cold water for two to three hours, rinse beans and then simmer in water (4 cups water to 1 cup beans) on the stove for about 30- 45 minutes. In Japanese cooking, they are used in desserts in the form of a sweetened paste called koshi-an or tsubushi-an. When adzukis are prepared with rice, the rice takes on a beautiful reddish-purple tint from the beans.

Almonds

Why: Research has shown that adding almonds to your diet helps keep weight off. They are a good afternoon alternative to quick, sugary foods, providing protein, magnesium, potassium, phosphorous, calcium and omega-9 (oleic acid). They also satisfy food cravings.

Where to buy it: At the grocery store

How much to eat: A ¼ cup daily as an afternoon snack will help satisfy hunger pangs.

Quick Tip: The almond is technically the seed of the fruit of the almond tree. Like its cousins the peach, cherry and apricot tree, it bears fruits with stone-like seeds (or pits). The seed of the almond fruit is what we refer to as the almond nut.

Quick Facts: A study published in the November 2003 issue of the *International Journal of Obesity and Related Metabolic Disorders* reported that an almond-enriched low calorie diet (which is high in monounsaturated fats), can help overweight individuals shed pounds more effectively than a low calorie diet high in complex carbohydrates. They found those eating almonds experienced a 62% greater reduction in their weight/BMI (body mass index), 50% greater reduction in waist circumference and 56% greater reduction in body fat compared to those on a low calorie high carbohydrate diet.

Bee Pollen

Why: Bee pollen's natural phenylalanine content acts as an appetite suppressant. Bee pollen helps build the immune system and provides energy for the entire body. It contains 35% protein, 55% carbohydrate, 2% fatty acids and 3% minerals and vitamins. It is high in B-complex and vitamins A, C, D and E and contains lecithin.

Where to buy it: Health food stores, in the refrigerated section. Bee pollen is actually many small granules similar to the size of grain of wheat or quinoa and is usually sold in a plastic container.

How much to take/eat: A common adult dosage of bee pollen granules is initially ⅛ to ¼ teaspoon once per day. The dosage is gradually increased to 1 to 2 teaspoons one to three times per day. Adults suffering from allergies are best advised to start off with one to three granules daily, and then gradually increase to higher doses- typically over a period of one month or more. Some people feel more energized with very little bee pollen while others need more. By starting slowly you will discover how your body reacts to bee pollen.

Quick Facts: According to researchers at the Institute of Apiculture, Taranov, Russia: "Honeybee pollen is the richest source of vitamins found in nature in a single food. Even if bee pollen had none of its other vital ingredients, its content of rutin alone would justify taking at least 1 teaspoon daily for strengthening capillaries. Pollen is extremely rich in rutin and may have the highest content of any source, plus it provides a high content of the nucleics RNA (ribonucleic acid) and DNA (deoxyribonucleic acid)."

Buckwheat

Why: The nutritional uniqueness of buckwheat is the quality of protein it contains. It offers all essential amino acids (nine proteins that the body cannot manufacture) in good proportions, making it closer to being a "complete" protein than any other plant source. This is a great complex carbohydrate, slowing down sugar cravings (low glycemic) and is a rich source of B vitamins, phosphorus, potassium, iron and calcium.

Where to buy it: At the grocery store or health food market.

How much to eat: A ½ cup equals 10 grams for protein, 8 grams of fiber and only 284 nutrient-dense calories.

Quick Facts: When researchers followed almost 36,000 Iowa women over a six-year long study of the effects of whole grains and the incidence of diabetes, they found that women who consumed an average of three servings of whole grains daily had a 21% lower risk of diabetes compared to those who ate one serving per week.

 Quick Tip: Many people think that buckwheat is a cereal grain. It's actually a fruit seed related to rhubarb and sorrel, making it a suitable substitute for grains for people who are sensitive to wheat (or other grains that contain protein glutens).

Figs

Why: Figs help satisfy your sweet tooth while providing an excellent source of minerals. They actually have the highest overall mineral content of all common fruits. A ¼ cup provides 244 mg of potassium, 53 mg of calcium and 1.2 mg of iron. Potassium, a trace mineral, balances water in the body, is important for building muscle and metabolizing protein and carbohydrates–all important factors for weight management and metabolism.

Where to buy it: At the grocery store or health food market–either fresh or dried.

How much to eat: One fresh fig is about 37 calories and a ¼ cup dried figs offers about 93 calories. Because figs are sweet-tasting and nutritious, they make a great afternoon snack with almonds.

Quick Facts: Research performed by the University of Scranton has determined that dried figs have a polyphenol content ranging from 4 to 50 times higher than other fruits. Polyphenols provide much of the flavor, color, and taste to fruits, vegetables, seeds, and other parts of the plants. As a dietary source of biologically active compounds, they have been linked to the reduced risk of cardiovascular disease, cancer and other degenerative diseases. Polyphenols have been associated with their antioxidant, antibacterial, anti-inflammatory, and anti-allergenic properties.

Green Superfood Drinks

Why: These functional food drinks are packed with nutrients from grasses, blue green algae and herbs that are nutrient-dense Superfoods. Many green drinks help improve metabolism, help balance blood sugar levels and give you natural energy getting you off the recliner and out for a walk. They are high in antioxidants, proving to be important in managing weight loss and Syndrome X. *(See Syndrome X paragraphs later in this chapter for details.)*

Where to buy it: Health food stores and some progressive supermarkets.

How much to take: Follow the recommended directions.

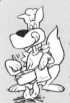

Quick Recipe
Meal Replacement Shake

- 1 Tbls high quality superfood drink
- 2 Tbls ground flax seed
- 1 Tbls lecithin granules
- 1 Tbls nutritional yeast
- ⅓ cup frozen berries

- ⅓ cup frozen shelled soybeans
- 2 Tbls plain yogurt
- ½ tsp of cinnamon
- ½ tsp of cooking chocolate–optional

Combine all the ingredients in a blender until smooth. Serve immediately after blending while the mixture still has a bubbly, milkshake-like consistency.

Salad Greens

Why: You can eat 2 cups of spinach leaves, 10 slices of cucumber, one medium tomato and a ¼ cup grated carrot for a whopping total of 67 calories! And you're getting the enzymes you need to help digest your food, fiber to keep things moving and antioxidants that keep your body feeling and looking young. Vegetables and fruits are among the best foods to maintain your weight!

Calories per Cup:

- **Shredded romaine** = 8 calories
- **Raw asparagus** = 27 calories
- **Raw broccoli** = 31 calories
- **Chopped cabbage** = 21 calories
- **Chopped carrots** = 52 calories
- **Celery** = 15 calories

- **Dandelion greens** = 25 calories
- **Raw mushrooms** = 15 calories
- **Onions** = 67 calories
- **Bell pepper** = 30 calories
- **Radishes** = 19 calories
- **Watercress** = 9 calories

A large salad topped with a good olive oil, balsamic vinegar dressing will satisfy and build energy.

Where to buy it: In the fresh produce section of the grocery store.

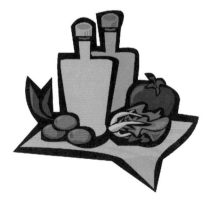

How much to eat: Eat at least one big salad a day, preferably for dinner.

Quick Tip 1: Choose a low fat, low sugar salad dressing. Blending frozen or fresh blueberries or strawberries with balsamic vinegar is slightly sweet and tangy and is a great substitute for store-bought salad dressing. Add olive oil or walnut oil for a great heart-healthy, weight-managing salad your shape will love.

Quick Tip 2: Extras: Add ¼ cup feta cheese (99 calories) or ¼ cup non-fat mozzarella cheese (42 calories) to your salad. A ¼ cup low fat Swiss cheese is only 59 calories and ½ cup of skinless, roasted chicken breast adds only 115 calories.

Sea Vegetables

Why: Sea vegetables are especially high in minerals, containing large quantities of calcium, phosphorous, magnesium, iron, iodine, folic acid, riboflavin and pantothenic acid. These iodine rich vegetables help keep your thyroid functioning, sometimes acting like a regulator, thyroid function is partly responsible for the metabolism. If you think you may have a low thyroid, getting iodine by way of Superfoods is the way to go.

There are thousands of types of sea vegetables that are classified into categories by color known either as brown, red or green sea vegetables. Each is unique, having a distinct shape, taste and texture. Some of the most popular types:

- **Nori** *(no·ri)*: Dark purple-black color that turns phosphorescent green when toasted; famous for its role in making sushi rolls.
- **Kelp:** Light brown to dark green in color–often available in flake form. Kelp is nature's richest source of iodine, a component of the thyroid hormones thyroxine (T4) and triiodothyronine (T3).
- **Hijiki** *(hi·ji·ki)*: Looks like small strands of black wiry pasta with a strong flavor.
- **Kombu** *(kom·bu)*: Very dark in color and generally sold in strips or sheets; often used as a flavoring for soups.
- **Wakame** *(wa·ka·me)*: Similar to kombu, most commonly used to make Japanese miso soup.
- **Arame** *(ar·a·me)*: This lacy, wiry sea vegetable is sweeter and milder in taste than many others.
- **Dulse:** Soft, chewy texture and reddish-brown in color.

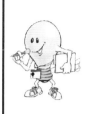

Quick Tip: Thyroid cells are the only cells in the body which can absorb iodine. The thyroid gland takes iodine (found in many foods) and converts it into thyroid hormones: thyroxine (T4) and triiodothyronine (T3). These thyroid cells combine iodine and the amino acid tyrosine to make T3 and T4. These are then released into the blood stream and are transported throughout the body where they control metabolism (conversion of oxygen and calories to energy). Every cell in the body depends upon thyroid hormones for regulation of their metabolism.

Where to buy it: Asian markets and some health food stores. Sea vegetables are sold in different forms. Look for sea vegetables sold in tightly-sealed packages. Avoid those showing evidence of excessive moisture.

How much to eat: Eat 3 to 4 ½ cup servings a week.

Snapper Fish

Why: Snapper is a great source of protein–4 ounces provide 29 grams of protein, 145 calories and less than 1 gram of saturated fat. The combined nutrients found in snapper make it an outstanding food for stabilizing blood sugar. It contains omega-3 fatty acids, protein, and B complex vitamins, which are all involved in blood sugar balancing keeping you from the urge to raid the refrigerator. Snapper is also a superb source of selenium, providing 56 mcg in 4 ounces. Selenium plays an important role in the body's enzyme function helping to metabolize food. It is also an important antioxidant that works to reduce the levels of damaging free radicals in the body–recently found to be connected with weight loss.

Where to buy it: In the fresh fish section or frozen seafood area of the grocery store.

How much to eat: Eating 4 ounces of fish, four to five times a week is most beneficial for weight management. You can trade off other fish such as salmon, tuna and small white fish throughout the week.

Quick Tip: There are about 185 species of snapper worldwide, and all belong to the family of fish called Lutjanidae. The largest red snapper ever caught was 50 pounds!

Sweet Potato

Why: Dubbed the "anti-diabetic" food, sweet potatoes have this label because of recent animal studies in which sweet potato helped stabilize blood sugar levels and lowered insulin resistance. This root vegetable is an excellent source of vitamin A (in the form of beta-carotene), a very good source of vitamin C and manganese, and a good source of copper, dietary fiber, vitamin B6, potassium and iron.

Quick Tip: Insulin resistance is a problem caused when cells don't respond to the hormone insulin, which normally acts as a key "unlocking" the cell to allow sugar to pass from the blood into the cell. When the body becomes insulin resistant we often carry more weight around the stomach area, and it's harder to keep the weight off.

Where to buy it: At the grocery store.

How much to eat: One medium sweet potato contains 135 to 155 calories. Eating sweet potatoes instead of russet potatoes will also satisfy your urges for sweets. You can eat ½ a potato daily if you like!

Watermelon

Why: With only 46 calories per cup, watermelon is an excellent source of potassium and vitamins A, C and B6. It contains 92% water and has no cholesterol and virtually no fat. Watermelon's lycopene content is close to that of tomatoes. Lycopene is a powerful antioxidant that helps protect cells and other structures in the body from oxygen damage. It's been linked in human research to the protection of DNA (our genetic material) inside of white blood cells.

Where to buy it: At the grocery store in the fresh produce section.

How much to eat: When you're in the mood to have something sweet, make it 1 cup (or even 2 cups) of watermelon.

Quick Facts: Watermelon is a vegetable, related to the cucumber, pumpkin and squash families.

Quick Recipe
Watermelon Gazpacho
(a mildly spicy refreshing soup)

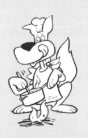

- 8 cups cubed, seeded watermelon
- ½ cup finely chopped onion
- ½ cup finely chopped green pepper
- 2 tsp fresh (if possible) basil
- ½ tsp salt
- ¼ tsp coarsely ground pepper
- ½ tsp chili powder
- 1 Tbls cider vinegar

In blender, puree watermelon with ¼ cup of onion and green pepper; pour into large mixing bowl. Stir in remaining ingredients (the other ¼ cup of onion and pepper). Refrigerate, covered, at least one hour to blend flavors. Makes 4 to 6 servings.

Wild Rice

Why: Wild rice is very low in fat and high in fiber. In addition, it has nearly twice the protein of other types of rice and it is loaded with B vitamins, folate, niacin, thiamin, iron, phosphorus, zinc and magnesium. These nutrients keep your body functioning correctly, burning up calories. Its chewy texture and nutty flavor is also very satisfying.

Where to buy it: At the grocery store.

How much to eat: One cup contains 166 calories, 7 grams of protein and a low glycemic index. Mixing wild rice with brown rice results in a milder taste. Wild rice complements dishes with fruits, nuts, meats, poultry and fish. Eating ½ cup to 1 cup daily will give you brain energy and keep you feeling satisfied.

 Quick Tip 1: Unlike its white and brown counterparts, wild rice, once cooked, expands three to four times its original size. A 6 ounce package of raw, wild rice yields four, ¾-cup servings.

 Quick Tip 2: To cook: place 1 cup wild rice in 3 cups boiling water or stock. Return to boil; reduce heat to slow boil and cover. Simmer for 40 to 50 minutes or until rice is tender. Drain any excess liquid. Fluff with fork and season to taste.

Water, Water, Water

Why: Drinking water is vital in maintaining weight loss and increasing metabolism. A report from *The Journal of Clinical Endocrinology and Metabolism* suggests that drinking sufficient water may actually increase the metabolic rate, or the rate at which we burn calories. Studies show that thirst and hunger sensations are triggered together. If there is a slight dehydration (and the body is really craving fluid), the thirst mechanism can be mistaken for hunger. The health benefits of drinking water include regulating appetite, increasing metabolism, boosting energy levels, less water retention and helping release toxic waste products from the body.

Where to buy it: This incredible liquid is found right in your own house (or you can have it delivered).

How much to drink: It may be helpful to portion out your daily water intake in the morning. Using plastic water containers, measure out at least ½ your body weight in ounces. Here's how: i.e., 150 pounds divided in half = 75 pounds. Next, convert that to ounces = 75 ounces/day. A medium sized bottle of water is approximately 25 ounces. So you should drink three of those each day. Drink at least this amount of water daily, if you want to feel even better–drink more!

Quick Tip 1: When you drink all the water your body needs, you will very quickly notice a decrease in your appetite, possibly as soon as the first day! Anyone serious about becoming leaner and healthier must drink water. If you're doing everything else right and still not seeing results, water may just be the missing link.

Quick Tip 2: Try a slice of lemon or lime in water to help maintain a good pH balance and improve liver function.

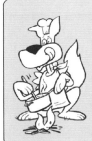

Quick Recipe

Spice up your water by making a peppermint-green tea blend that's refreshing either hot or cold. This combination also gives you energy as it soothes the digestive tract. If you don't need the caffeine found in green tea, steep the tea for less than five minutes.

Quick Facts: In a University of North Carolina study, researchers reviewed eating habits of nearly 5,000 people and found that those who drank about seven cups of water daily ate nearly 200 fewer calories than those who drank less than a glass a day. Water avoiders tend to scarf down more high-fat foods than hydrators and guzzle twice as many soft drinks.

———— Herbs ————

Cinnamon

Why: According to cellular and molecular studies at the University of California, Santa Barbara, Iowa State University and the U.S. Department of Agriculture, cinnamon is an insulin substitute in Type II diabetes. Cinnamon itself has insulin-like activity, increasing the effectiveness of insulin. Cinnamon also has a bio-active component that has the potential to prevent or overcome diabetes. It also increases vitality, balances energy, improves the digestion of fruits, milk, and other dairy products and helps reduce bloating and gas.

Where to buy it: At the grocery store. If you have access to purchasing on line, you can purchase cinnamon in bulk very inexpensively. My favorite is www.mountainroseherbs.com.

How much to take/eat: One of the easiest things you can do to improve blood sugar and increase insulin is add up to a ½ teaspoon of cinnamon to your cereal, green drink or protein drink daily.

129

Quick Tip 1: Cinnamon is particularly good for people who tend to have a hot upper body and a cooler lower body.

Quick Tip 2: More than 170 million people worldwide suffer from diabetes.

Quick Facts: A study published in *Diabetes Care* examined 60 people with Type II diabetes. Thirty men and 30 women, with an average age of 52, were divided into six groups: groups one, two, and three consumed one, three, or six grams of cinnamon daily, respectively, and groups four, five, and six were given placebo capsules corresponding to the number of capsules given to the other groups. After 40 days, all three groups taking cinnamon had a reduced fasting blood glucose ranging from 18 to 29%, triglycerides 23 to 30%, LDL cholesterol 7 to 27%, and total cholesterol 12–26%.

Quick Tip 3: Cinnamon also comes in an essential oil. This is not recommended for consumption as the active insulin-enhancing compounds in cinnamon are found in the dry powder form, not the oil.

A Dysfunctional Metabolism

Understanding metabolism is crucial to maintaining the new you. The truth is metabolism is regulated by what we eat. The term metabolism refers to the way that your body processes and uses the food you eat. Rather than saying "faster" or "slower" metabolism, it's most accurate to describe metabolism as efficient or functional versus inefficient or dysfunctional.

Metabolism is affected by three components:
1. Basal metabolism: 60–65 % of the calories you eat daily are spent keeping you alive and providing basic energy for life support, even if you do nothing but sit and watch TV.
2. Physical activity: 25% of your calories go to movement and physical activity.
3. Thermic effect of food: About 10% of calories are spent processing the food you eat. If you eat 2,000 calories per day, you use up 200 calories through eating and digestion alone.

Simply put, to maintain weight you need to ensure that the calories going in are equal to the calories going out. Embracing a little hunger can be a positive thing, signaling to your brain that your stomach is not being overindulged. Give your body what it needs to be strong, but not so much that you're looking for a place to take a nap.

Several factors affect metabolism:

Hypothyroidism or too little thyroid hormone is also called underactive thyroid. If you suspect you have hypothyroidism, get tested by your doctor. Symptoms of hypothyroidism include weight gain, constipation, dry skin and sensitivity to the cold.

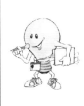 **Quick Tip:** For a Hypothyroidism Home Test, you will need a thermometer (it can't be digital; it must be a mercury thermometer). For four to five days before you get out of bed in the morning, take your temperature at your underarm; yes, your armpit. Leave the thermometer there for five minutes, and then record the results. If the results are consistently less than 96 degrees you may be hypothyroid, which will affect your metabolism (not to mention your energy levels and your enthusiasm for Living It!). Be sure to verify your findings with your doctor.

Genetics. Some people can eat anything and remain slim, while others swear that by simply looking at food they gain weight. Genetically–low metabolism can be elevated through muscle building activities. Adding weight-bearing or resistance exercise training is one of the only ways to increase basal metabolism.

 Quick Tip: Muscle cells are up to eight times more metabolically active than fat cells, and muscle burns more calories than fat.

Dehydration. Dehydration contributes to inefficient metabolism by affecting body temperature. When dehydrated, the body temperature drops slightly, causing it to store fat as a way to help raise or maintain its temperature.

Foods. Eating proteins versus simple carbohydrates and fats increases the thermic effect and the resting metabolic rate as much as two to three times. Complex, high-fiber carbohydrates, like vegetables and whole grains, burn more calories than simple carbs. Eating quality protein, high-fiber fruits and vegetables, grains and beans also increases thermic metabolism. Recent research adds that antioxidants found in vegetables, fruits, legumes and herbs are an important component of weight management and metabolism.

———— Secrets to "Living-It" ————

Maintaining your new-found weight loss is doable once you understand what you need to eat, how often and the best times to indulge.

1. Eat four to five small meals a day. This helps your body raise its metabolic thermic effect, stops the high and lows of blood glucose balancing and helps eliminate the starving syndrome.

2. Balance your intake of good carbs, proteins and healthy fats.

3. Consume the same amount of calories that you use up in a day. Here's a way to approximate that number:

   For adult males: Multiply the body weight by 10; add double the body weight to this value. For example for a 150 lb male, 1,500 + (2 x 150) = 1,800 calories a day.

   For adult females: Multiply body weight by 10; add the body weight to this value. For example a 120 lb female, 1,200 + 120 = 1,320 calories per day.

4. Enjoy your life! If you want a piece of cake at your aunt's birthday party, have it; then continue smart eating afterward. Don't beat yourself up–just add an extra 15 minutes to your exercise routine later that day and be extra careful on your food choices.

Next, let's calculate your daily food intake:

The 40-30-30 Basic Wellness Plan

Divide food groups into these percentages:
- 40% calories: good carbohydrates
- 30% calories: protein
- 30% calories: healthy fats

A 2,000 calorie day will help maintain your weight:
- 800 calories: carbohydrates (200 grams)
- 600 calories: proteins (150 grams)
- 600 calories: healthy fats (63 grams)

 Quick Tip: If you'd like to lose more weight, here's how to calculate the amount of calories to consume daily: Multiply 10 times your current weight, but **don't** add your body weight as we did previously (i.e. if you weigh 150 pounds, your total calorie intake would be 1,500. This calculation does not apply if you are severely overweight).

Quick Fact: In 2003, a 10-year US study found that pleasant, floral-spice perfume makes women appear 10 pounds lighter in the eyes of the opposite sex. A perfume diet may be the next big thing!

——— Exercise Your Right to Exercise! ———

Moving your body is vital to "living-it" as it burns calories, resets the metabolic set point, decreases hunger and increases metabolism all day and evening (for up to two to eight hours after exercising). Exercise is the most effective way to keep your metabolism from slowing down. A general guideline is to do aerobics three days a week and lift weights two to three days a week. It's important to also have a rest day, allowing the muscles to rest and repair.

Research shows that exercise for fat loss is most effective between noon and 8 p.m. But the best time to exercise is whenever you can fit it into your schedule! Be aware of the way you feel during and after exercise–involvement in the moment is key to staying with and benefitting from it.

Aerobics

Working at 60-75% of your maximum heart rate will help burn fat for energy and increase the metabolism of fat. You will be burning a greater percentage of fat calories. This requires working more slowly for a longer period of time. Start with at least ½ hour of aerobics every other day and work up to one hour every other day.

Calculating the Heart Rate Maintaining a 60-75% Heart Rate

Example: 220 minus your age (i.e., 220 – 36 = 184)

184 x .60 = 110

184 x .75 = 138

To make sure you're staying in this range, take your heart rate at the hardest level of your workout. Count your heart beats for 10 seconds. In the example above, your heart rate should be between 18 and 23 (110 and 138 divided by 6). If it's not within those levels, adjust your workout accordingly.

Weight Lifting

Weight lifting releases even more endorphins than aerobics. Gentle, but progressive resistance training will help put on lean muscle mass. But remember: muscle tissue is dense and weighs more than fat tissue. In a weight loss of six pounds of fat, with a gain of two pounds of lean muscle mass, the scale would show no weight loss, although you'll look and feel better. This is a good reason why you should not weigh yourself for the first two months of starting weight training. Judge your success instead by the way your clothes fit.

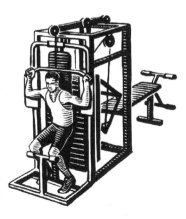

133

Quick Facts: *The Journal of Clinical Endocrinology and Metabolism* reported that when you don't get enough sleep your blood level of leptin—a hormone that suppresses your appetite—drops. When the level drops, your appetite will increase for high-calorie, high-carbohydrate foods. To help maintain your leptin levels, and reduce your urge to overeat, get six to eight hours of sleep a night.

The Hidden Dangers (and Hidden Names) of Sugar

There has been a rise in Type II diabetes in very young children that has never been seen before. It's estimated that by the age of 40, one out of ten Americans will be diagnosed with Type II diabetes. Diabetes leads to heart disease, macular degeneration and circulatory problems in the body.

Quick Tip 1: Manufacturers love to put sugar in processed food. It's cheap and it makes food taste better. Sugar is an added ingredient in many processed foods, health bars and health drinks. But it's not always easy to identify the sugar ingredients. The easier ones are sucrose, fructose, maple syrup and molasses. The trickier ones to look for are dextrose, turbinado, amazake, sorbitol, carob powder and high fructose corn syrup.

Quick Tip 2: **How much sugar is in your food?** To determine how much sugar is in a serving of any food, check the nutrition label; sugar is listed in grams. Divide the number of grams by four to get the actual teaspoons of sugar per serving (i.e., 12 grams would equal 3 teaspoons of sugar). Alcohol sugar is somewhat better than regular sugar but it is still sugar. If the ingredient label says 12 grams of alcohol sugar, divide that by two then divide by four and you will have your sugar content (i.e., 12 grams of alcohol sugar is equal to 1.5 teaspoons of sugar). Warning: carefully read the labels of fat free products. Many use more sugar than the product with a normal fat content.

———— Syndrome X ————

Syndrome X has been linked to rising levels of obesity and declines in physical activity. It's diagnosed when a person has three or more of the following conditions: abdominal obesity, high triglyceride levels, low HDL ("healthy" lipoprotein) cholesterol levels, high blood pressure and high fasting blood sugar levels. People who have syndrome X are at greater risk of developing Type II diabetes and heart disease. Sufferers are also more likely to die prematurely from heart disease and other causes. Syndrome X, as well as Type II diabetes, pre-diabetes and obesity, all can be viewed as different facets of the same disease—having the same underlying dietary, lifestyle and genetic causes.

The Causes of Syndrome X

The human body is not designed to handle the amount of refined sugar, salt, saturated fats and other harmful food compounds that many people in the United States and other "Western" cultures consume–especially for those who live a sedentary lifestyle. The result, metabolic syndrome emerges–elevated insulin levels, obesity, elevated blood cholesterol and triglycerides and high blood pressure.

Under normal conditions, a hormone known as insulin allows blood sugar to move into the cells of the body, where it is used to produce energy. Resistance occurs when the cells resist the action of insulin and the glucose cannot pass into the cells. When this happens, the pancreas must produce more insulin to maintain normal blood glucose levels. Although people with syndrome X have higher levels of glucose in their blood, it is still within the normal range, and they are not considered diabetic.

Slowing Down Syndrome X

It is well established that the safest, most effective and preferred way to reduce insulin resistance in overweight and obese people is through weight loss and increased physical activity. Adding soluble dietary fiber like oat bran, nuts, barley, flax seed and fruits and vegetables helps improve many of the symptoms of Syndrome X.

- 30% of the American population is insulin resistant. Some studies estimate as high as 50%.
- 20% of children under the age of 17 are thought to be insulin resistant.
- 90% of Type II diabetics are overweight.
- 50% of Type II diabetics die from heart disease.

Chapter 8

. . . .

Superfoods for Ligaments, Joints and Bones

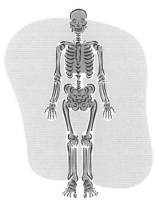

Sore, creaky joints aren't just a sign of age and over use. That popping and crackling you hear as you hobble out of bed in the morning could be signs of osteoporosis (porous bones) and osteoarthritis. Osteoporosis is a thinning of the bone tissue and loss of bone density over time. Osteoarthritis is the deterioration of the joint cartilage (softer parts of bones that cushion their connections to each other). These two diseases afflict many people simultaneously, and nutrition plays a definitive role in preventing or alleviating both of these painful conditions.

Many people resort to pain-killing substances and anti-inflammatories to reduce the pain caused by poorly healed torn ligaments and cartilage, creaky and inflamed joints and weak bones. Though bone, ligament and cartilage health begins early in life, it's not too late to affect relief naturally. Superfoods can actually stop deterioration as they help create stronger healthier bones and joints. Adding these Superfoods to your daily diet helps reverse the affects of agonizing bone and joint diseases.

Quick Facts: The World Health Organization calls osteoporosis its biggest global healthcare problem with aging populations, exacerbated by obesity. Obesity increases inflammation throughout the body, including in bones where it significantly contributes to osteoporosis. Today, a woman's lifetime risk of an osteoporotic fracture is 30-40%, and even men face about a 13% risk. When calcium levels in the blood drop below normal, calcium is taken from bone, unless replaced through diet.

Bone Tips

- ✓ The knees provide stable support for the body. They also allow the legs to bend and straighten. Both flexibility and stability are needed to stand, walk, run, crouch, jump, and turn. Other parts of the body help the knees do their job. These are:
  - o Bones
  - o Cartilage
  - o Muscles
  - o Ligaments
  - o Tendons
  - o *If any of these parts are injured, the knee may not function properly.*
- ✓ Both bone and cartilage are living tissue, constantly forming (bone formation) and breaking down (bone resorption).
- ✓ Researchers estimate about 20% of American women over the age of 50 have osteoporosis.
- ✓ Bones contain 99% of the body's total calcium, essential for bone health. The remaining 1% is in the blood, needed for nerve conduction, muscle contraction and blood clotting.
- ✓ Antioxidants may slow the rate of joint deterioration in osteoarthritis patients. In particular, vitamin E has been shown to reduce the symptoms of osteoarthritis.
- ✓ Joint diseases account for more than half of all chronic conditions in the elderly.
- ✓ In the United States, musculoskeletal conditions cost up to $254 billion per year in medical care and loss.
- ✓ According to the American Academy of Orthopedic Surgeons, about four million people in the United States seek medical care each year for shoulder sprain, strain, dislocation or other related problems.

Superfoods for Ligaments, Joints and Bones

Chickpeas (aka garbanzo beans)

Why: Chickpeas are an excellent source of bone-building nutrients. A ½ cup contains 105 mg calcium, 115 mg magnesium, 875 mg potassium, 19 grams protein, zinc, iron, copper, selenium, folate, vitamin K and B6, and chickpeas are low in sodium. When you get your protein from garbanzos, you also get the blood sugar-stabilizing and heart-health benefits of the soluble fiber provided by these versatile legumes.

Where to buy it: At the grocery store, either dried or canned.

How much to eat: Five to six servings weekly would be ideal.

Quick Facts: At every stage of life, an individual's bone mass and bone strength status are a product of the balance between *bone resorption* (mediated by osteoclasts) and new *bone formation* (mediated by osteoblasts). When the two processes are in balance, bone mass and strength are constant. When bone resorption becomes dominant, osteoporosis occurs.

Quick Recipe

This high protein, vegetarian salad is very quick and easy to prepare. In fact it can be made in just 15 minutes from start to finish, and kept for several days in the refrigerator, getting more flavorful as it marinates. Using fresh herbs and a small amount extra virgin olive oil makes this a healthier, flavorful salad than many of those with high fat dressings.

- 1 15-oz can garbanzo beans, drained and rinsed
- ⅔ cup chopped green onions
- 1 medium clove of pressed garlic
- 1 medium ripe tomato, or ¼ cup chopped sun dried tomatoes
- 3 medium celery stalks, chopped coarse
- 3 Tbsp fresh lemon juice
- 2½ Tbsp chopped fresh mint
- 3 Tbsp chopped fresh parsley or cilantro
- Extra virgin olive oil to taste
- ¼ cup feta cheese (optional)

Mix all ingredients together, except feta cheese-sprinkle on top when serving. The recipe makes four servings.

Dandelion

Why: Dandelion leaves are loaded with bone-building, cartilage-strengthening nutrients. One cup has 147 mg calcium, 25 mg magnesium, 244 potassium, 2.1 grams protein, zinc, iron, silica, copper, selenium, folate and vitamins B6 and K. Dandelion greens are also great for the digestive tract.

Where to buy it: Many markets now carry this healthy green in the produce section.

How much to eat: If you want to aid bone density, add dandelion to your salads as often as you can!

139

Quick Tip: The leaves are a rich source of vitamin A and also contain vitamins B, C and D. It's bitter compounds help stimulate digestion, increase bile production in the liver and bile flow from the gallbladder. The increase in bile flow helps improve fat metabolism, including cholesterol.

Figs

Why: Figs have the highest overall mineral content of all common fruits. Just a ¼ cup provides 244 mg of potassium, 53 mg of calcium, 25 mg magnesium and 1.2 mg of iron. Potassium has been found to be an important nutrient for bone and cartilage formation, plus it's important for building muscle and metabolizing protein and carbohydrates. Figs are also a good source of zinc, selenium, vitamins B6, K and folate.

Where to buy it: At the grocery store or health food market—either fresh or dried.

How much to eat: One fresh fig is about 37 calories and a ¼ cup dried figs contains about 93 calories. Because figs are sweet-tasting and nutritious, they make a great afternoon snack with almonds.

Kale

Why: Kale is a great source of calcium (calcium is one of the key nutrients needed to make healthy bones). Dairy products are a heavily-promoted source of this nutrient. But unlike dairy products, kale is not a highly allergenic food, nor does it contain any saturated fat. Plus, a cup of kale supplies 93.6 mg of calcium for only 36.4 calories. In contrast, one cup of 2% cow's milk provides 296.7 mg of calcium, but the cost is high: that same cup contains 121 calories and 14.6% of the day's suggested limit on saturated fat. On the other hand, one cup of kale provides 28 mg magnesium, 299 mg potassium, vitamins K, B6 and folate as well as the minerals zinc, copper, selenium and iron.

Where to buy it: In the produce section of the grocery store.

How much to eat: Kale is great added to salads. Eat ½ to one cup daily to help strengthen bones and ligaments.

Quick Tip: Kale is a leafy, green vegetable that belongs to the Brassica family, a group of vegetables including cabbage, collards and Brussels sprouts, that have gained recent widespread attention due to their health-promoting, sulfur-containing phytochemicals.

Quick Recipe

Sauté kale with fresh chopped garlic, pine nuts, a little lemon juice and olive oil.

Milk (*non fat, dry*)

Why: Milk remains the best dietary source of calcium for two reasons: the lactose (milk sugar) found naturally in milk and the vitamin D added to it enhances calcium absorption through the gut. In infants, lactose nearly doubles the rate of calcium absorption. In just ½ cup of non-fat dry milk powder you get a whopping 754 mg calcium, 66 mg magnesium, 1076 mg potassium, 22 grams protein, zinc, selenium, B6, B12, folate and iron. I like non-fat dry milk because you can add just ¼ cup to your daily shake in the morning and afternoon and get a healthy dose of calcium!

Where to buy it: At the grocery store.

How much to drink: It's been found that consuming calcium in smaller doses throughout the day aids in absorption. Drink a ¼ - ½ cup in the morning, afternoon and before you go to bed.

Quick Tip 1: Dairy products provide calcium that is readily absorbed, but calcium absorption may be negatively affected if the foods are eaten with wheat bran. This means when you add calcium-fortified milk to your wheat bran cereal in the morning, you've just negated the calcium bone-building properties!

Quick Tip 2: Substitute non-fat, dry milk in recipes that call for milk to get added calcium benefits.

Quick Facts: The bone growth and body growth of children, teenagers and young adults is called *bone modeling*–when the body adds length, width and height to the bones. During the bone modeling stage, 100% of the bone surface is active. After the bone modeling stage, *bone remodeling* begins–we maintain bone growth associated with fixed adult bone mass. In bone remodeling, only about 20% of the bone surface is active. During this phase, older bone tissue is destroyed (bone resorption) and replaced by new bone tissue (bone formation) in a continuous process.

Olive Oil

Why: Olive oil has bone-sparing effects. Its polyphenols, oleuropein and hydroxytyrosol greatly lessen the inflammation-mediated bone loss involved in osteoporosis. France's National Institute for Agricultural Research team found that people eating a traditional Mediterranean diet were less likely to develop osteoporosis.

Where to buy it: Purchase extra virgin olive oil at your grocery store.

How much to eat: Consuming just 1 to 2 tablespoons a day is beneficial. Substitute olive oil for butter when craving a slice of bread and butter. Add a few drops of balsamic vinegar to the oil for a better taste.

Quick Facts: Olive oil is the only vegetable oil that can be created simply by pressing the raw material, olives. The quality of the oil depends on the amount of processing involved. Extra virgin olive oil is the least processed and is considered nutritionally best.

Parmesan Cheese

Why: Parmesan cheese can be added to many dishes and just ¼ cup provides 344 mg of calcium, 12 mg of magnesium, 26 mg of potassium, 10 grams protein as well as zinc, selenium, folate, B6, B12 and vitamin K. These nutrients are vital to bone formation and ligament flexibility and strength. For as little as a ¼ cup, parmesan cheese is a powerful Superfood.

Where to buy it: In the cheese section of the grocery store, or you can buy it already grated.

How much to eat: Add a ¼ cup to your salad, or as a topping on sautéed turnip greens, four to five times a week. Alternating between bone, ligament and joint Superfoods throughout the week will give you variety. Eat at least one serving per day.

Sardines

Why: Sardines contain all of the essential nutrients to aid in inflammation of creaky joints and in bone formation. Consuming just a ½ can (1.9 ounces) of sardines gives you 175 mg calcium, 18 mg magnesium, 182 mg potassium, 11 grams protein as well as zinc, copper, iron, selenium, B12 and folate. Sardines are also a great source of omega-3 with 238 mg in 1.9 ounces. Omega-3s are known for their anti-inflammatory action, giving relief to sore, achy joints!

Where to buy it: At the grocery store.

How much to eat: Eat one ½ can of sardines four to five times a week.

Quick Recipe
Curried Sardine Spread

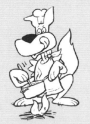

- 1 can boned, skinned sardines packed in olive oil
- 1 cup ricotta cheese
- 1 Tbsp curry powder
- ¼ cup fresh chopped parsley
- 2 Tbsp capers, drained
- 1 tsp lemon juice

Drain oil from sardines and discard tails. Combine sardines with remaining ingredients in a food processor and process to a coarse, "spreadable" form. Serve with crisp crackers.

Soy Foods

Why: Many soy foods, such as tofu, fortified soymilk, tempeh, soybeans and textured vegetable protein are excellent sources of highly bioavailable calcium (approximately 30 to 40% of the calcium is absorbed). Soy protein favorably affects calcium metabolism, relative to other high quality proteins, and it's been found that soybean isoflavones may directly inhibit bone resorption (breaking down). Incorporating soyfoods into the diet is one easy way to help reduce risk of developing osteoporosis. Just a ½ cup of shelled, raw soybeans provides 204 mg calcium, 83 mg magnesium, 793 mg potassium, 16 grams protein along with zinc, silica, copper, selenium, iron, folate and vitamins A and C.

Where to buy it: Look in the frozen vegetable section of the grocery store for soy beans. Tofu is found in the produce, dairy or deli sections of the grocery store. Edamame is the soybean still in its pod (or purchase shelled soybeans).

How much to eat: Substitute tofu for meat or poultry dishes four to five times per week. Shelled beans can be lightly steamed for five minutes and added to salads.

Quick Tip: There are three basic types of tofu: Firm (good for stir-frying, soups or on the grill); Soft (great for recipes that call for blended tofu or in Oriental soups); or Silken (this form of tofu is a creamy, custard-like tofu, and best used for pureed or blended dishes).

Quick Facts: Soyfoods contain isoflavones, compounds that may directly inhibit bone resorption. The isoflavones are similar in chemical structure to estrogen, which promotes bone health. They are nearly identical in structure to the drug ipriflavone, which inhibits bone resorption and has been used successfully in both Asia and Europe to treat osteoporosis. To be maximally effective, ipriflavone has to be metabolized. One of the metabaolites of ipriflavone is daidzein, one of the two primary isoflavones in soybeans. There is now animal data indicating that genistein, the other primary soybean isoflavone, directly inhibits bone resorption. Human studies examining the effects of soyfoods are under way.

Swiss Cheese, Low Fat

Why: Snacking on one slice of Swiss cheese gives you 269 mg of calcium, 24 mg of magnesium, 31 mg of potassium, 8 grams protein as well as zinc, selenium and B12. Eating one slice of low fat Swiss cheese three times a day will give you the nutrients needed to strengthen joints and bone for a total of 150 calories!

Where to buy it: At the grocery store in the cheese section.

How much to eat: Eat one to two slices daily with another serving of calcium-rich Superfoods daily for the best bone and joint protection.

Quick Tip: Start your day with a Swiss cheese omelet made with omega-3 eggs and chopped kale. For lunch have a salad with dandelion greens, sprinkled with parmesan cheese and for dinner create a tofu stir fry with your favorite vegetables. Eating these three meals will give you all the calcium/magnesium and nutrients for stronger bones, more cushioned joints and connective tissue nutrients for flexible ligaments.

Turnip Greens

Why: If you're concerned about rheumatoid arthritis, turnip greens are a good food to add to your shopping list. The beta-carotene in turnip greens provides vitamin A (low levels of vitamin A are associated with rheumatoid arthritis). Vitamin A also helps the body to produce and maintain healthy membranes, including the synovial membrane that lines our joints. Plus, per cup, you get 105 mg calcium, 17 mg magnesium, 163 mg potassium as well as zinc, copper, iron, selenium, folate and vitamin K. Turnip greens also have vitamins C and E, found to help with reduced inflammation. Turnip greens provide the collagen building blocks for ligament repair and minerals for bone formation.

Where to buy it: At the grocery store.

How much to eat: Eat one cup daily or in a mix with other calcium-rich foods.

> *Quick Tip:* Turnip greens are the leaves of the turnip plant, better known for its tasty root. Turnip belongs to the Cruciferae family, a cousin to other health-protective giants including kale, collards, cabbage and broccoli. For basic turnip green preparation, wash the leaves and fold each leaf in half with the top side of the green folded inward. Cut along the stem and remove. Keep the leaves whole if you plan to cook the greens for a long time (in soups).

Whey Powder

Why: Adding whey powder to your morning or afternoon shake can be beneficial to your bone health. Whey is one of the few protein powders with significant calcium. Adding two tablespoons of whey powder will provide 112 mg calcium, 12 mg magnesium, 126 mg potassium, 6 grams of protein, zinc and selenium.

Where to buy it: At health food stores, drug stores and progressive markets.

How much to eat: Two tablespoons per day in your shake, or mixed with water.

Yogurt *(low fat, plain)*

Why: We've all heard the benefits of yogurt and they are true! Yogurt is a great source of essential nutrients for bone and joint health. Eight ounces contain 208 mg calcium, 19 mg magnesium, 251 mg of potassium, 12 grams of protein, zinc and selenium. Warning: yogurt contains a relatively high amount of sugar (that same 8 ounce serving contains 16 grams of sugar–or 4 teaspoons). If you're watching sugar intake, eat yogurt sparingly.

Where to buy it: At the grocery store in the dairy section. I recommend *Stonyfield Yogurt.* It contains six active cultures, providing a wide array of beneficial bacteria. When purchasing yogurt look for the words "live acidophilus," otherwise you're not getting the probiotics benefits.

How much to eat: Because of the high sugar content, alternate yogurt with other sources of calcium, magnesium and vitamin D. Eat one 8 ounce serving daily.

> *Quick Facts:* Sugar may also deplete our bodies of calcium. In one study, administering 100 grams (about 25 teaspoons) of sugar (sucrose) to healthy volunteers caused a significant increase in the urinary excretion of calcium. When the same amount of sugar was given to people with a history of calcium oxalate kidney stones or to their relatives, the increase in calcium excretion was even greater. Because 99% of the body's total calcium is in our bones, this increase in calcium excretion most likely reflects a leaching of calcium from bone.

Water, Water, Water

Why: One of the easiest ways to begin the reversal of connective tissue damage is to drink more water. By weight, connective tissue is comprised of 60 to 80% water. Water and proteoglycans (mortar-like substances made from protein and sugar that are the building blocks of cartilage) enables ligaments to be strong and somewhat flexible. Dehydration is a major reason joints stiffen and cause pain. Dehydration especially affects the cartilage lining in bones, joints and discs, and is a contributing factor to degenerated discs. As the collagen fibers wind around each other, they begin to contract and the molecules become shorter and tighter. Water is squeezed out (like squeezing a sponge), which also causes shrinkage. As the millions of collagen fibers lose water and shrink, the ends of the ligament will be slowly pulled together and elasticity decreases.

Where to buy it: This incredible liquid is found right in your own home or at the grocery store.

How much to drink: Drink at least ½ your body weight in ounces daily, i.e., 150 pounds divided in half = 75 pounds; next, convert that to ounces = 75 ounces/day. A medium sized bottle of water is approximately 25 ounces. So you should drink **three** of those each day.

 Quick Tip: Keep in mind that thirst is an indicator of dehydration; it is *not* an early warning sign. By the time you feel thirsty, you may already be dehydrated. Other symptoms of dehydration include dizziness and lightheadedness, having a dry or sticky mouth and/or producing less and darker urine.

Quick Facts: Preliminary research indicates that 8 to 10 glasses of water a day could significantly ease back and joint pain for up to 80% of sufferers.

Herbs for Inflammation

Boswellia

Why: A German research review suggested gum resin from boswellia may help with inflammatory diseases including rheumatoid arthritis (RA) and colitis. One such clinical study involved 30 patients with knee osteoarthritis (OA) who received boswellia extract or placebo for eight weeks. All patients receiving boswellia reported decreases in knee pain and swelling, increases in knee flexion and an increase in walking distance. The treatment showed only minor gastrointestinal adverse effects.

Where to buy it: At health food stores.

How much to take: Follow the recommended dosage on the bottle.

Quick Facts: Also called Indian frankincense, boswellia is the gum resin from the bark of a tree that grows abundantly in the hills of India. Known for its anti-inflammatory effects, this resin has historically been used in traditional Indian medicine to support joint health. Laboratory studies suggest it may also help block the release of an enzyme that breaks down cartilage. One well–conducted clinical trial in 2003 revealed that patients taking 1,000 mg of supplemental boswellia daily experienced easier movement, less swelling, and a better ability to bend their knees, compared to the period during which they were given a placebo.

Ginger Root

Why: Ginger contains very potent anti-inflammatory compounds called gingerols. These substances are believed to explain why so many people with osteoarthritis or rheumatoid arthritis experience reductions in their pain levels and improvements in their mobility when they consume ginger regularly. In two clinical studies involving patients who responded to conventional drugs and those who didn't, physicians found that 75% of arthritis patients and 100% of patients with muscular discomfort experienced relief of pain and/or swelling when taking ginger root. Ginger root is an excellent antioxidant that is believed to also help bring down inflammation.

Where to buy it: At the grocery store in the fresh produce section.

How much to drink: There are a few ways to get your "gingerols"; making a tea from the fresh root is easy. Thinly slice a ½ inch ginger piece and place in eight to 10 ounces of water, bring water to a boil, then reduce temperature and simmer about 15 minutes. I like to make a big pot and keep it in the refrigerator. Drink three to four cups a day–hot, warm or cold!

> *Quick Facts:* A study published in the February 2005 issue of the *Journal of Alternative and Complementary Medicine* sheds light on the mechanisms of action that underlie ginger's anti-inflammatory effectiveness. In this research, ginger was shown to suppress the pro-inflammatory compounds produced by the cells comprising the synovial lining of the joints.

Spices *(tarragon, oregano, cumin seed, thyme and parsley)*

Why: All these spices are good sources of calcium, magnesium and antioxidants. Adding a teaspoon here and there while cooking provides flavor for your dishes, as well as important nutrients for joints, bones and ligaments. Plus, these spices are loaded with antioxidants, many known to help reduce inflammation.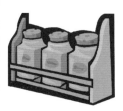

Where to buy it: At the grocery store or on line at www.mountainrose.com.

How much to eat: Add a teaspoon to your meals when cooking.

Turmeric

Why: Turmeric's combination of antioxidant and anti-inflammatory effects explains why many people with joint disease find relief when using this spice. In a recent study of patients with rheumatoid arthritis, turmeric was compared to prescription medication and over the counter NSAIDS, it showed comparable improvements in morning stiffness, lengthened walking time and reduced joint swelling.

Where to buy it: At the grocery store or Indian market.

How much to eat: Add ¼ to ½ teaspoon of the powder in a tea, two to three times daily between meals. To make the tea, place a ½ teaspoon of powder into 1 cup of boiling water, infuse for five minutes, strain and drink. You can add ginger or cardamom to add flavor and speed-up absorption.

No Bones About It, Nutrients Are the Way to Go

Boron

Boron is a trace mineral required to convert estrogen and vitamin D to their most active forms. Studies have shown that boron provides protection against osteoporosis and reproduces many of the positive effects of estrogen therapy in postmenopausal women. One study of postmenopausal women also concluded that supplementation with three mg of boron per day reduced urinary calcium excretion by 44%. Estrogen levels drop after menopause causing osteoclasts to become more sensitive to parathyroid hormone, which signals them to break down bone.

The best dietary source of boron is fruits and vegetables and as such, a diet deficient in fruits and vegetables is most likely a diet deficient in boron.

 Quick Tip: The U.S. Second National Health and Nutrition Examination survey found that less than 10% of Americans meet the minimum recommendation of two fruit and three vegetable servings per day, and 51% of Americans eat only one serving of vegetables per day.

Calcium

Many factors affect the supply and demand of calcium in the human body. The developmental stage of the individual dictates how much calcium is needed to build and maintain strong bones as well as the development of a growing fetus in pregnant women. Intestinal function also plays a role in calcium levels. The body is able to alter the level of absorption of calcium from food. Individuals with low calcium intake are able to absorb a greater fraction of intestinal calcium than those who chronically ingest higher amounts. As the quantity of calcium increases, the percentage that is absorbed decreases. For that reason, consuming no more that 400-600 mg of calcium at one time is most beneficial.

Studies confirm consuming calcium throughout the day from foods is better absorbed than from pills. Eating a varied diet is the best way to absorb calcium. And then only 20 to 30% of calcium in the average diet is absorbed, because it binds to some fiber, phytate (found in unleavened grain products) or oxalate (found in some green vegetables) in the intestine.

 Quick Tip 1: It's been found that supplemental calcium carbonate is not well absorbed. If you're taking a supplement, calcium citrate or calcium malate are the best bioavailable for the body.

> **Quick Tip 2:** Another great benefit of calcium is that it limits the absorption of lead and exposure to lead stored in the skeleton which can be mobilized by demineralization.

- **Absorption Inhibited**

  Factors which inhibit calcium absorption and may contribute to calcium loss are: aluminum (foods cooked in aluminum cookware), aluminum foil and antacids containing aluminum, digestive disorders and high levels of magnesium. Oxylates (a chemical that is found in sweet potatoes, dried beans, rhubarb and spinach), and concentrated forms of phytic acid (found in wheat bran and dried beans) inhibit calcium absorption. So what does this mean? When you combine wheat bran with milk (for calcium) your body won't be able to absorb the calcium because the phytic acid found in the wheat bran will block its absorption; the same happens when you eat spinach and drink milk. Without the minerals magnesium, potassium, phosphorous, iron, silica and vitamins D and K, (important codependent nutrients) calcium will also not be absorbed.

- **Calcium Excretion**

  Aside from the issue of dietary calcium absorption, there is the issue of calcium excretion. According to the *Journal of Nutrition,* 1990, protein consumption below 200 gm/day (the average protein intake around 75 grams daily), will equate to an approximate 1.2 mg of calcium loss (via the urine) per protein gram intake. This means if you consume the average 75 grams of protein daily, you will excrete 90 mg of calcium. Also, alcohol, phosphates (in soft drinks and meats) and sugar will increase calcium excretion.

> **Quick Tip 1:** The pre-pubescent and adolescent years are critical ones in forming a strong skeleton. This strong skeleton can be developed through engaging in physical activity and a healthy diet, preventing the development of or decreasing the degree of osteoporosis in later years. Peak bone mass is achieved around the age of 30. During the peak bone development years (9 through 17), this age group drinks more soft drinks than milk, thereby limiting calcium intake and contributing to calcium excretion during their formative years.

Quick Facts: Consumption of excessive amounts of alcohol is a known risk factor for osteoporosis. In a study of 96 chronic male alcoholics, ages 24 to 62, 47% had osteoporosis. Among those under the age of 40, 31% had osteoporosis. Although a similar study has not been done on women, it is likely that drinking too much alcohol will also promote osteoporosis in women. The effect of moderate alcohol consumption on bone health is not known.

EFAs

EFAs have been shown to increase calcium absorption from the gut (in part by enhancing the effects of vitamin D), reduce urinary excretion of calcium, increase calcium that is deposited in the bone and improve the strength of bone. New research provides evidence that omega-3 fatty acids can significantly decrease bone turnover rates. In women, these beneficial omega-3 fats work with estrogen to stimulate bone mineral deposits and slow the rate of bone breakdown.

EFAs are also beneficial for inflammation and pain. In a report in the *Surg Neurol*, April 2006, written by Department of Neurological Surgery, University of Pittsburgh Medical Center, Pittsburgh, Penna., it was found that of 250 patients, 78% percent were taking 1200 mg and 22% were taking 2,400 mg of EFAs. Fifty-nine percent discontinued taking their prescription NSAID medications for pain; 60% stated that their overall pain was improved and 60% stated that their joint pain had improved. An overwhelming 80% were satisfied with their improvement, and 88% stated they would continue to take the fish oil. There were no significant side effects reported.

Glucosamine Sulfate/ Chrondrotin

These are often found in combination in cartilage. Research from the Division of Rheumatology, University of Utah School of Medicine, Salt Lake City, as reported in the *New England Journal of Medicine,* February, 2006 reported a great deal of research on the mechanisms of action and efficacy of these two ingredients in osteoarthritis. For patients with moderate-to-severe pain, the rate of response was significantly higher than those with mild pain. The exploratory analyses suggest that the combination of glucosamine and chondroitin sulfate may be effective for people with moderate-to-severe knee pain. It's also been found that these two nutrients work for some and not for others, but there is no clear reason why. If you do not feel results by the fourth to sixth month, then you will not receive benefits from these two supplements. Both these supplements can be purchased at drug stores, vitamin shops and some grocery stores.

Iron

When you think of ways to build strong and healthy bones, most people immediately mention calcium. However, new research indicates that iron also makes a difference in your bone health.

151

A combined study at the Universities of Arizona and Arkansas found that postmenopausal women who consumed at least 18 milligrams of iron per day had the greatest bone mineral density levels. The role of iron in bone density may be linked to its role in the production of collagen, a key component of our bones. Researchers also found that iron's benefits may be tied to calcium consumption in the range of 800 to 1,200 milligrams per day. It appears that a balanced intake of iron and calcium has the best benefit for bone health.

Magnesium

The highest amounts of magnesium are found in the skeleton. The next highest is in the muscle tissues and the remainder is found in other tissues and fluids. Magnesium is essential for energy production, protein formation and cellular replication (e.g., DNA, RNA). It's as important as calcium and phosphorus. Magnesium works with calcium to metabolize it, in muscle contraction and relaxation (calcium-contraction, magnesium-relaxation). It also works with vitamin D, potassium and other minerals, and it helps reduce blood pressure, reduce vascular spasm and improve heart function.

 Quick Tip: Caution: high doses of supplemental zinc and high protein intake interfere with magnesium absorption.

Phosphorous

Calcium and phosphorus are "co-dependent" nutrients affecting the health of bones and soft tissues. When they are out of balance, bone disease can develop. Phosphate makes up more than half the mass of bone mineral. Thus, the diet needs to have sufficient phosphorus in order to have healthy bones.

The balance of calcium and phosphorus can especially affect women over 60 whose diets often contain less than the recommended dietary allowance of 700 mg of phosphorus. For these women, the usual calcium supplement (calcium carbonate) may block most of the absorption of phosphorus. If this happens, the calcium won't do much good as bone mineral consists of both calcium and phosphorus.

 Quick Tip: Excessive levels of phosphorus in the diet can also cause problems, especially if the kidneys are not removing excess phosphorus from the bloodstream. When phosphorus is too high, the body takes calcium out of the bones to bind with the phosphorus and remove it from the blood. The subsequent calcium loss results in porous and brittle bones.

Potassium

Potassium is important to help retain calcium as it appears to counteract the increased urinary calcium loss caused by high-salt intake (10 g of salt per day will subtract about 70 mg per day from retained calcium by increasing calcium losses in urine). Aim for 4,000 mg of extra potassium from your diet–it will add 60 mg per day to retained calcium and reduce calcium losses.

Potassium is also known as an electrolyte that maintains the electrical charge of the cell–critical for nerve and muscle function and contraction. Potassium needs replenishing after hard exercise and profuse sweating. Low potassium results in low levels of stored glycogen or muscle fuel, and potassium deficiency can result in fatigue and muscle weakness.

Quick Facts: A clinical trial of 60 postmenopausal women on high-salt diets found that those whose daily intake of potassium was equal to the amount found in seven to eight servings of fruits and vegetables had a lower calcium loss than those whose diets were not supplemented with potassium.

Proteins

Proteins are essential in our diets to build tissue during growth, protein repairs and replaces tissue throughout the life cycle. It is also needed for fracture healing. Interestingly, too much protein intake and not enough calcium along with vitamin D can cause calcium loss. Protein also increases the body's need for calcium by increasing calcium *excretion.* As protein is burned for energy, it produces a chemical called sulfate, which the body excretes through the kidneys. Sulfate increases the excretion of calcium.

Quick Facts: A report in the *American Journal of Clinical Nutrition,* 2005, reported a three-year study suggesting that bone mineral density (BMD) may actually benefit from high-protein diets, *only* when recommended dietary allowance of calcium and vitamin D were met.

Selenium

At an American College of Rheumatology Annual Meeting in San Diego, 2005, investigators from the University of North Carolina reported that low levels of selenium were strongly linked to arthritis of the knee. The risk for knee osteoarthritis was 40% lower in those with the highest selenium stores compared to those with lowest. In

153

addition, the chance of having severe disease was nearly halved in this group. And in this study, some of the benefits of having adequate selenium stores were even stronger for African-Americans. These researchers will now study whether selenium affects knee cartilage or whether the benefits come from selenium's antioxidant role.

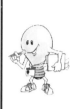 ***Quick Tip***: Bones that meet at joints have soft caps of cartilage at the ends, and years of bending and rubbing can start to wear these caps down. Osteoarthritis (OA) is common, affecting about 20 million people. OA is a "wear and tear" disease and becomes more common as people get older. Those symptoms range from mild stiffness to severe pain. Most people develop the condition to some degree in at least one joint by age 60. Fingers, knees and hips are most often affected. The frequency of OA starts to rise after age 50 among men, and after age 40 among women, and symptoms tend to get more severe as people age.

Silica

Silica cross-links collagen strands to strengthen the connective tissue matrix of bone. The presence of concentrated silica at calcification sites in growing bone seem to indicate that sufficient levels of silicon are required for bone remodeling. Silica has a physiological role in bone formation. Harvard and Tufts Universities reported that dietary silica intake is positively associated with bone mineral density (BMD), at least for men and pre-menopausal women. Bone and cartilage abnormalities are associated with a reduction in matrix components, resulting in the establishment of a requirement for silica in collagen formation.

Abnormalities in bone formation can be induced in animals by keeping them on a low-silicon diet. Edith M. Carlisle, Ph.D., discovered that calcium and vitamin D alone are not sufficient for bone growth, density, strength and flexibility. Other minerals, including traces of silica, are needed to strengthen bones and increase production of collagen, the tough, flexible connective tissue that binds everything together. Carlisle established that a deficiency in dietary silica is an important–yet little considered–risk factor for osteoporosis and osteopenia.

Horsetail (equisetum arvense) is an excellent natural source of silica. It's also rich in calcium and several other minerals needed to rebuild injured tissue and is helpful in the healing of arthritis. Silica's many benefits include improved cell metabolism, stimulated cell formation, inhibited aging process in tissues, strengthened weak connective tissue and improved structure and function. It also increases the elasticity and firmness of blood vessels, making them less likely to develop atherosclerosis. It aids in reducing inflammation reactions and has been found to stimulate the immune system to fight off disease-causing invaders:bacteria, viruses and toxins.

Silica needs other minerals to aid its uptake: boron, magnesium, manganese and potassium each helps make use of dietary silica. Iron and phosphorous, in particular, are needed for our bodies to help assimilate this trace mineral.

Vitamin A

Vitamin A is important for healthy bones. However, too much vitamin A has been linked to bone loss and an increase in the risk of hip fracture. Scientists believe that excessive amounts of vitamin A may trigger an increase in osteoclasts, the cells that break down bone. They also believe that too much vitamin A may interfere with vitamin D, which plays an important role in preserving bone. It's better to get extra beta carotene from foods and let the body naturally regulate how much of this precursor is converted to vitamin A. It's highly unlikely that a person could take in enough beta carotene to produce a toxic amount of vitamin A, because when the body has enough vitamin A, it stops making it.

Vitamin K

Found to play a significant role in bone formation, vitamin K improves bone health. Human intervention studies have demonstrated that vitamin K not only increases bone mineral density in osteoporotic people, but also actually reduces fracture rates. Further, there is evidence in human intervention studies that vitamins K and D, a classic in bone metabolism, works synergistically on bone density.

Vitamin D

Vitamin D has a positive effect on calcium balance as it increases calcium absorption in the gastrointestinal tract. Vitamin D does not directly cause the increased absorption, but rather begins a series of events which affect intestinal absorption of calcium. The most readily available source of vitamin D is exposure to direct sunlight, exposure for as little as 15 minutes a day on arms, legs and face has a positive 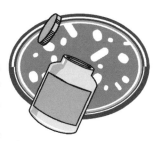 effect. For those who find it hard to go into the sun daily, obtain vitamin D from fatty fish, cod liver oil capsules or liquid, eggs, liver, butter or fortified foods such as milk and multivitamins.

Vitamin B6, Folic Acid and Vitamin B12

All three of these vitamins interact with the enzymes and chemicals in complex ways, affecting the levels of homocysteine in our body. Homocysteine (found in higher levels in postmenopausal women) obstructs collagen cross-linking, which results in poor bone matrix and osteoporosis.

Zinc

Found with its highest concentration in muscles (65%), zinc is also found in red and white blood cells, bone, skin, liver, kidneys, pancreas, eye retina, in the male prostate gland and sperm. It helps make cell membranes strong and is important in neurological development. Zinc is an important component of the nutritional package for rheumatoid arthritis, as it's been found to fight inflammation. Several studies have shown that people who have rheumatoid arthritis have low blood levels of zinc, often associated with high levels of inflammatory biochemicals in the blood.

Zinc absorption is decreased by drinking tea and coffee. Its absorption can also be decreased if eaten with foods that are high in phytic acid (found in fiber). It joins the phytic acid and forms zinc-phytate, which is not absorbed. High intakes of calcium, iron and copper may also limit zinc absorption. It's best to get zinc from food; taking a supplement that is not balanced with copper can create biological imbalances.

Exercise for Bone, Joint and Muscle Health

You probably know that exercising can help build up your muscles. But did you know it also improves the strength of your bones? It does! Activities such as dancing, playing tennis, gymnastics, and even walking keep your bones strong. Doing a variety of activities will give you the best benefits. Joints are made to move. When we rest our body too long, we slowly weaken muscles. As a result, the tendons that attach muscle to bone become less elastic. To a person with arthritis, this adds up to more pain and stiffness. Regular exercise helps the muscles become stronger; the tendons more limber, and exercise creates a reduction in pain and stiffness. Most people begin to notice improvements within two months, and some feel better almost immediately.

It's been found that weight-bearing exercise (one in which your feet and legs bear the brunt of your body weight) is great for building up bone density. The reason is that muscle pulls on bone, which in return builds bone. The best exercises for building bone are weightlifting, jogging, hiking, stair climbing, step aerobics, dancing, racquet sports and other activities that require your muscles to work against gravity. Exercises such as swimming or a slow casual walk are not the best exercises for building bone, but any exercise is better than none. If you already have osteoporosis, start exercising; it's never too late!

Thirty minutes of weight-bearing exercise daily benefits not only your bones, but improves heart health, muscle strength, coordination and balance. It's not required that you do 30 minutes at once; it's equally beneficial to do 10 minutes at a time.

For the best benefit to your bone health, combine several different weight-bearing exercises. As strength increases, add more weight (or resistance) rather than increasing repetitions. Combine weight-bearing and resistance exercises with aerobic exercises to help improve your overall health. Add more physical activity to your day. Take the stairs versus the elevator; park farther way from the building; and walk to your co-worker's office for a face-to-face conversation rather than sending an email.

- **Osteoarthritis** sufferers also benefit from exercise by stimulating the blood flow to the cartilage that cushions joints. Unlike most tissues in the body, cartilage doesn't receive nutrients from the bloodstream. Instead, it gets its nourishment from fluid (called synovial fluid) in the joints. When a joint moves, the fluid sloshes around, giving the cartilage a healthy dose of oxygen and other vital substances. As an added bonus, regular exercise encourages the body to produce extra synovial fluid.

- **Arthritis**. For arthritis sufferers, stretching and range-of-motion exercises (slowly moving the joints through their full range), strength training, as well as aerobics are most beneficial. Also, according to the Arthritis Foundation, yoga provides relief for arthritis pain. Yoga is an ancient discipline based on the Hindu practice of mind-body unity. It combines stretching, strength training, and range-of-motion exercises with mental and spiritual training; most forms include breathing and meditation techniques. A small, randomized, controlled study published in the *Journal of Rheumatology* in 1994 indicated that yoga significantly improved tenderness, pain and range of motion in the fingers among subjects with osteoarthritis of the hands. Another study that year in the *British Journal of Rheumatology* demonstrated that yoga was useful in treating rheumatoid arthritis.

Chapter 9

·····································

Superfoods for Radiant Good Health, Skin, Hair and Nails

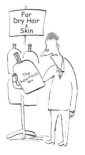

Many people have a healthy glow at 30, but how do you stay shining at 50? There is one thing every possessor of true beauty has in common–**health**. It's a sure bet that anyone who can turn heads at 50 is healthy on the inside. Good nutrition plays a major role in determining how we feel on the inside and how we look, move and even how we relate to the world on the outside. Certain minerals and vitamins have a direct influence on the functioning of blood vessels, cell regeneration, waste removal and in balancing the delicate collagen matrix that keeps skin, hair and nails in peak health. A balanced diet is essential because our skin, hair and nails are the *last* parts of the body to get nutrients from our food. Nutrients first go to the heart, brain, lungs and other vital organs. Whatever is leftover goes to the skin, hair and nails. Getting plenty of the vital minerals, vitamins and other nutrients is the only way to ensure hair, skin and nails get their much-needed share–and to keep heads turning in admiration.

Superfoods for Skin, Hair and Nails

Avocados

Why: Leading the Superfoods for skin, avocados contain over eight of the vital nutrients needed to produce new skin cells, help prevent skin cancer and provide EFAs that keep the skin looking dewy and soft. Also, this wonderful fruit is high in vitamins A, C and E–important antioxidants for aging skin.

Where to buy it: At the grocery store. Look in the fresh produce section or in the freezer section. Also look for guacamole containing the least ingredients and without added preservatives.

How much to eat: Eat ⅓ to ½ of a medium size avocado three to four times a week.

 Quick Tip: Avocados vary in weight from 8 ounces to 3 pounds, depending upon the variety. A ripe, ready-to-eat avocado is slightly soft, but should have no dark sunken spots or cracks. If the avocado has a slight neck (rather than rounded on top), it was probably tree ripened and will have better flavor. To ripen quickly, place in a brown paper bag with an apple; it will be ready to eat in a couple of days.

Asparagus

Why: This member of the lily family is a rich source of the minerals silica, zinc, copper and selenium—each important for the formation of fibroblasts that create collagen in the dermis layer of the skin. Collagen is a protein that forms the basic substance of body structures including the skin, connective tissue, cartilage and tendons. Also, asparagus has a high amount of bioavailable silica, necessary for hair and nail production. Asparagus also contains the vital nutrients vitamins A, B, C and K.

Where to buy it: At the grocery store in the fresh produce section. If it's not in season, look in the frozen foods section.

How much to eat: Eat 1 cup three to four times a week.

 Quick Tip 1: The spears we buy in the store are actually the shoots from an underground crown. It takes up to three years for crowns to develop enough to begin producing shoots, but once they do, they can produce for up to 20 years.

 Quick Tip 2: Lightly steaming asparagus for one to two minutes brings out the color and nutrients. Don't over cook—all vegetables have a delicate balance of nutrients and enzymes; over-cooking decreases nutrients significantly.

 Quick Tip 3: Creams that contain collagen **don't** actually give your skin more elasticity. However, they **do** help your skin retain moisture.

Braeburn Apples

Why: They are rich in vitamin C, potassium, fiber and antioxidants such as ellagic acid and flavonoids. This superstar also has a high amount of quercetin which helps inhibit allergy responses (and allergic hives).

> *Quick Facts:* It's been found that the phenols in the skin of apples have a hefty dose of UV-B protection, according to a study published in the August 2003 issue of *The Journal of Experimental Botany*. The next time you plan to spend time in the sun, consider taking along a few apples to snack on.

Where to buy it: At the grocery store.

How much to eat? Taking a sun-filled vacation to Hawaii or the Caribbean? Eat one to two apples a day for sun protection. Remember to bring the sun screen also!

> *Quick Fact:* Apples are a part of the rose family, like pears. They are originally thought to be from Europe and south Asia, and there are over 7,000 varieties.

Brazil Nuts, Cashews, Pistachio Nuts and Sunflower Seeds

Why: These are all excellent sources of the minerals zinc and copper (essential nutrients for hair growth). Copper and zinc are found in large amounts in the hair follicle and are thought to enhance the production of the hair shaft and are necessary nutrients for collagen production and wound healing. Brazil nuts are also an excellent source of selenium, a powerful antioxidant that helps eliminate free radicals.

Where to buy it: At the grocery store.

How much to eat: Eating just two Brazil nuts daily or a ¼ cup to ⅓ cup of these nuts or seeds as an afternoon snack helps cut carbohydrate cravings for candy and soda.

> *Quick Tip:* Roasted or raw—both are okay, but beware of salted nuts. We typically don't need the added sodium.

Brussels Sprouts

Why: Brussels sprouts are an excellent source of vitamin C, the body's primary water-soluble antioxidant. Vitamin C is essential for collagen manufacturing. In addition, a cup of Brussels sprouts contains a whopping 1,122 IU of vitamin A plus 669 IU of beta-carotene, both of which play important roles in defending the body against infection and promoting supple, glowing skin.

Where to buy it: At the grocery store.

How much to eat: The FDA recommends 8 to 10 servings of vegetables and fruits daily. Making Brussels sprouts one of those servings will help keep your skin glowing.

Quick Facts: Sulforaphane, an active compound found in Brassica family of vegetables, has been shown to boost liver and skin cells' detoxifying abilities. Now, new research, conducted at Johns Hopkins University and published in the November 2005 issue of *Cancer Letters,* indicates sulforaphane can help repair sun-damaged skin.

 Quick Tip: Plant phytochemicals found in Brussels sprouts enhance the activity of the body's natural defense systems to protect against disease, including cancer. Brussels sprouts are members of the brassica family and therefore are kin to broccoli and cabbage.

Green Peas

Why: Part of the legume family, green peas are packed with skin-rejuvenating nutrients such as zinc and copper for the development of collagen, and vitamins A, B and C for skin cell formation. Green peas also contain a very high amount of lutein and zeaxanthin, antioxidants specific to eye health. So why include green peas in a skin, hairs and nails chapter? Well, the better your eyesight, the less you squint and that translates to fewer wrinkles around your eyes!

Where to buy it: At the grocery store in the frozen section–only 5% of farmed peas are available fresh from the market.

How much to eat: Eat 1 cup, three to four times a week.

 Quick Tip: The less water you use when cooking peas, the less vitamin C is lost. Steaming peas helps to preserve this essential vitamin.

Kiwi

Why: Kiwi fruit is an excellent source of vitamin C, an important nutrient in collagen formation in the skin. Kiwi is also a good source of two of the most important fat-soluble antioxidants, vitamins E and A. Vitamin A is provided in the form of beta-carotene. This combination of both fat–and water-soluble antioxidants allows kiwi to provide free radical protection on all fronts.

Where to buy it: At the grocery store.

How much to eat? One kiwi fruit constitutes one of the recommended daily 8 to 10 servings of vegetables and fruits.

Quick Tip 1: Eat kiwi soon after cutting into it, as it contains enzymes that act as a food tenderizer, making the fruit soft very quickly. When adding kiwi to a fruit salad, do so at the last minute so the other fruits don't become soggy.

Quick Tip 2: If your skin is dry and flaky, it may be a sign of vitamin A deficiency.

Omega-3 Enriched Eggs

Why: Omega-3 enriched eggs come from hens fed a special diet containing 10-20% ground flaxseed. These eggs are the same as the traditional eggs except they have higher levels of polyunsaturated fatty acid called omega-3. Eggs are one of nature's most nutrient-dense foods and their protein helps our cells manufacture keratin for our hair and nails. Omega-3 enriched eggs are a good source of low-cost, high-quality protein, providing 5.5 to 6 grams of protein (11.1% of the daily value for protein) in one egg. Eggs also are an excellent source of B vitamins, selenium, vitamin D and K. Enriched omega-3 eggs give you the needed EFAs (essential fatty acids) to help prevent dry, brittle nails. It also helps our sebaceous glands provide oil to our hair and elasticity to our skin.

Where to buy it: Some grocery stores carry these Superfood eggs, but if you can't find them there, visit a health food store.

How much to eat: Eat 1 enriched egg daily or at least four to five enriched eggs weekly.

Quick Tip: Make a vegetable omelet with spinach, bell peppers, tomatoes and onions to give you the added nutrients for hair and nails.

Purple Grape Juice

Why: Many of the health benefits of grape seeds can be obtained by consuming purple grape juice, as the seeds and skin are not removed during its manufacturing. Approximately 33% of the therapeutic compounds in grapes are found in the seeds. This Superfood—or super drink—contains Oligomeric Proanthocyanidins (OPCs) to stimulate the proliferation of hair follicles and convert the hair growth cycle from a resting phase to a growth phase.

Where to buy it: At the grocery store.

How much to drink: Drink a 6 ounce glass daily, or look for a green drink containing grape seed extract.

Quick Tip: Be sure you get 100% Concord grape juice with *no* added sugar. Beware—many frozen juices add sugar. One six ounce glass serves as one of your daily 8 to 10 fruits and vegetables.

Soybeans & Tofu

Why: Considered to be one of the world's most nutrient-rich Superfoods (and the most widely researched, health-promoting foods around), soybeans are considered equal in protein quality to animal protein. Protein is essential to healthy skin, hair and nails. In addition to healthy protein, some of soybeans' nutritional high points include a good deal of easily-absorbed iron, magnesium and omega-3 fatty acids.

Where to buy it: Look in the frozen vegetable section of the grocery store for soy beans. Tofu is found in the produce, dairy or deli sections of the grocery store.

How much to eat: One cup of cooked soybeans is equal to 22 grams of protein. Substituting soybeans for red meat at least four to five times a week is great for overall health benefits.

 Quick Tip 1: Edamame is the soybean still in its pod. Gently steam soy beans for five minutes. They're yummy added to salads and soups.

 Quick Tip 2: There are three basic types of tofu: Firm (good for stir-frying, soups or on the grill); Soft (great for recipes that call for blended tofu or in Oriental soups); or Silken (this form of tofu is a creamy, custard-like tofu, best used for pureed or blended dishes).

Shrimp

Why: Shrimp are anything but small in their nutrient value. They are an excellent source of selenium and an unusually low-fat, low-calorie protein. Shrimp also contain vitamin D and the minerals zinc and copper, necessary nutrients for healing wounds.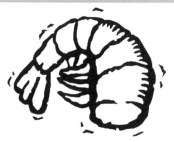

Where to buy it: At the grocery store, either fresh or frozen.

How much to eat: Eat 4 to 6 ounces, two to three times a week.

164

Quick Tip: The best way to thaw a block of shrimp is slowly, refrigerated for 24 to 48 hours. A quicker way is to run cold water over them. You can steam, boil, grill, deep-fry, sauté or stir-fry–just remember that shrimp cooks quickly. To see if it's properly cooked, hold the shrimp between your fingers and press it. You're looking for a slightly firm, but springy feel. If it feels soft and offers no resistance, the shrimp is undercooked. If the flesh is firm and does not spring back, it's overcooked.

Walnuts

Why: This delicious nut is an excellent source of omega-3 essential fatty acids which aids in reducing inflammatory skin diseases such as eczema and psoriasis. It also contains vitamins B, C and E and minerals zinc, copper and selenium necessary for skin cell production.

Where to buy it: At the grocery store.

How much to eat: Eat a ¼ cup of walnuts daily–or every other day.

 Quick Tip: Walnuts contain an antioxidant compound called ellagic acid that supports the immune system and is thought to offer several anti-cancer properties. Look for walnuts with no salt added to avoid the extra sodium.

Water

Why: Water, the priceless elixir of life, keeps our skin cells hydrated. Water also helps our body eliminate excess acid and toxins through the skin.

Where to buy it: This incredible liquid is found right in your own house! Of course, you can also purchase water at the grocery store.

How much to drink: Here's an easy way to figure out how much water you should drink each day: Drink at least ½ your body weight in ounces, i.e., 150 pounds divided in half = 75 pounds; next, convert that to ounces = 75 ounces/day. A medium sized bottle of water is approximately 25 ounces. So you should drink **three** of those each day.

Super Herbs for Skin, Hair and Nails

Equisetum Arvense *(horsetail herb)*

Why: Silica from horsetail is much more highly bio-available than purely mineral sources of silica due to the presence of flavonoids and other co-factors in the extract, which enhance silica's uptake. What was that? Think of silica from a bamboo plant–strong and flexible. That's what we want our hair and nails to be, right? Adding horsetail gives our bodies the added minerals for nail strength and hair growth. Silica is also an important element in collagen production and wound healing.

Where to buy it: Health food stores and some grocery stores. Equisetum is also available as a tea or supplement in capsule form.

How much to eat/take: If you prefer it in capsule form, take between 150 mg to 400 mg each day along with your calcium supplement. When making tea, add 1 teaspoon per 8 ounce cup of boiling water, let steep for 15 minutes, then drink.

Quick Facts: Edith M. Carlisle, Ph.D discovered that traces of silica are needed to strengthen bones and increase production of collagen, the tough, flexible connective tissue that binds everything together. Carlisle established that a deficiency in dietary silica is an important–yet little-considered–risk factor for osteoporosis and osteopenia. Horsetail's silica content increases the absorption of calcium, beneficial in hair and bone strength and is known to help detoxify the body of aluminum.

Red Clover

Why: Red clover is a great source of many nutrients including calcium, chromium, magnesium, niacin, phosphorus, potassium, thiamine and vitamin C. This powerful herb is known to be a great blood cleanser, keeping our skin glowing and free from blemishes. It is also thought to contain large amounts of isoflavones–polyphenols that mimic estrogen in the body.

Where to buy it: Health food store.

How much to eat/take? Red clover makes a delicious tea. Add 1 teaspoon of dried herb and blossom per cup of boiling water; let steep for ten minutes. Drink one to three cups per day.

> ***Quick Tip:*** Red clover is used traditionally as an ointment applied to the skin to treat conditions such as psoriasis, eczema and other rashes. It can be used externally as a hydrocortisone cream replacement for alleviating skin inflammations.

Nutrients for Radiant Good Health – Skin, Hair and Nails

Vitamins C and E

Both powerful antioxidants, vitamins C and E offset the effects of sun exposure. Vitamin C improves the integrity of collagen and increases its synthesis in the skin. Vitamin E increases the elimination of cellular waste through the skin, increases the growth of new skin cells and is thought to help improve blood circulation to the skin.

Vitamin A

Vitamin A contributes to the repair and the growth cycles of the skin.

B Vitamins

The B vitamins are essential for healthy hair, skin, nails, eyes and our liver function. Many of the B vitamins are directly related to the appearance of the skin. They help counteract dermatitis (itchy, scaly skin reaction) and keep the skin smooth and glowing. B vitamin, biotin regulates the secretion of sebum, counteracting the signs of dry skin and a sallow gray complexion. Vitamin B5 is required by the skin to synthesize protective fats that are essential to skin function. Additionally, foods rich in B vitamins supply energy to our cells, feeding the follicle and nail matrix.

> ***Quick Tip 1:*** During times of dieting or fasting it's easy to have B vitamin deficiencies. Because of their water-soluble nature, they're not stored in the body and therefore are excreted within a short time. If not replaced often, deficiencies result. Eating habits that include large amounts of refined and processed food, sugar, or alcohol also decrease the absorbency of B vitamins.

> ***Quick Tip 2:*** It's hard to take in too much B vitamins; our body excretes the excess.

Silica (*silicon*)

Silica is necessary for the production and healing of the skin by stimulating the activation of fibroblasts and elastin involved in the formation of collagen. It strengthens the dermal papillae of the hair follicles involved in hair growth and helps prevent hair loss. Silica is usually found in the outer layers or skin of foods. Unfortunately, silica is often the first to go during food processing.

Selenium

Selenium is a powerful antioxidant that plays a key role in skin cancer prevention.

Zinc and Copper

These important minerals help keep our skin looking moist. They are important in wound-healing and the development of collagen (responsible for the skin's elasticity). Copper and zinc are found in large amounts in the hair follicle and are thought to enhance the production of the hair shaft.

Protein

Required for the cells in the hair dermal papillae (follicle) and nail matrix to make keratin protein, protein is the primary substance of our nails and hair. We need essential amino acids (broken-down proteins) to supply our blood with the nutrients for the matrix and dermal papillae. Not eating enough protein will leave skin dull and weak and prone to imperfections. Skin blemishes can take longer to heal and you may find yourself more prone to unpleasant problems, like cold sores.

Essential Fatty Acids or EFAs

These EFAs are vital for our skin, hair and nails! EFAs maintain the oils in our hair, giving it shine. They also prevent our hair from becoming too dry, causing breakage. The nail bed, cuticle and skin around the nail require these beneficial nutrients too to keep them from becoming brittle and cracking.

Quick Tip: EFAs assist in improving eczema, psoriasis and other disorders of the skin. When the skin is properly nourished with EFAs, it becomes smoother, feels much softer and actually becomes less susceptible to infection. The skin ages more slowly and remains considerably more wrinkle-free for longer. In fact, with the presence of essential fatty acids, the skin becomes *radiant*.

The "Skinny"

- ✓ Skin makes up 15% of your body weight.
- ✓ The average adult has a surface area of skin between 15 to 20 square feet.
- ✓ Skin thickness varies from 2 to 3 mm ($\frac{1}{16}$ to $\frac{1}{8}$ inch).
- ✓ An average square inch of skin holds 650 sweat glands, 20 blood vessels and more than 1,000 nerve endings.

✓ Our skin pH is 4.5 acidic, protecting us from invasion of bacteria.
✓ We lose about 30,000 to 40,000 dead skin cells **every minute.**
✓ 95% of our epidermis cells are working to make new skin cells, the other 5% make melanin which gives skin its color.
✓ Skin is the largest organ in the body.

Skin: Read All About It

Our skin is not all about youthfulness; it's responsible for some major functions in our body. Skin:

- Protects our organs and tissues
- Eliminates excess salt, water, urea and toxins
- Regulates our body temperature
- Protects against harmful organisms
- Stores nutrients (fat cells)

There are three layers of skin: the epidermis, dermis and subcutaneous tissue.

- **The epidermis** is the outer layer of skin. Its thickness varies in different types of skin. The thinnest is on the eyelids at .05 mm and the thickest is on the palms and soles at 1.5 mm. The epidermis contains five layers. The bottom layer is where the divided cells push the already-formed cells into the higher layers. When they reach the top layer, they flatten and eventually die. Our top layer, the stratum corneum, is made of dead, flat skin cells that shed about every two weeks.

- **The dermis** is the layer of skin beneath the epidermis that consists of connective tissue and cushions the body from stress and strain. It also harbors many nerve endings that provide the sense of touch, heat and pain. The dermis contains the hair follicles, sweat glands, sebaceous glands and blood vessels. The blood vessels provide nourishment to the skin.

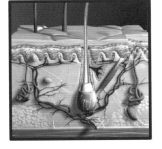

- **The subcutaneous layer** of the skin is below the dermis and is often called the hypodermis. It consists of adipose tissue (fat) and loose connective tissue that gives our body insulation and energy reserves.

Aging and Your Skin

Let's talk about the effects of aging on the largest organ in your body—your skin. About 70% of the dermal and epidermal skin layers are made of collagen fibers which form a network that makes healthy skin elastic and smooth.

As we age, the number of fibroblasts (a type of skin cell, ligaments and cartilage) starts to decline causing wrinkles, sagging skin and age spots. So how do we go about supplementing our aging body's need for fibroblast-friendly nutrients? Eating Superfoods high in silica is a good start. Silica (silicon) is a nutrient essential for the production of collagen, which in turn stimulates the activation of fibroblasts.

More Great Tips for Youthful Skin

Skin is the largest eliminative organ and plays a vital role in ridding the body of toxins and impurities. It has been estimated that the skin eliminates more than one pound of waste per day. Practiced for centuries, dry brushing the skin helps open the pores and stimulate circulation of the blood vessels and lymphatic system. Daily dry skin brushing is a great way to help retain that healthy, glowing skin without removing the protective mantle of acid and oils.

Saunas, steam baths, aroma-therapy baths and Epsom salt soaks are excellent ways to detoxify through the skin, dramatically increasing circulation and cleansing. Sweating brings toxins to the surface of the skin. If you don't have access to a sauna, you can exercise! Exercising enhances the body's natural detoxification process just as efficiently.

Quick Tip: Detoxification is essential for people with skin disorders. The liver is the major organ involved in many processes of detoxification, including the removal of toxins from our blood. The lungs bring the oxygen to the body and convert it to energy for the cells. The digestive system absorbs nutrients into the circulatory system to nourish the tissues and cells. Proper balance and function of the liver, lungs, and digestive system maintains healthy skin, thus your skin can benefit from all these detoxifications. For details on detoxifying, see the Superfoods for Internal Cleansing chapter.

Hair-Raising Truths

- ✓ Hair follicles are some of the most active cells in the body, dividing rapidly. As such they are *extremely* sensitive to what you eat.
- ✓ Approximately 35 new hairs grow each day.

✓ The average scalp contains about 100,000 hairs.
✓ Hair often grows more quickly in winter than in summer.
✓ Hair thickness is determined by the size of the follicles and how many of them line our scalp. Large follicles produce thick hairs. Small follicles produce thin hairs.
✓ Follicles that are round in cross-section produce straight hair. Those out of which curly hair grows are oval. Very tightly coiled hair is due to the nearly flat, ribbon-like structure of the follicles. (See diagram)
✓ The average life of a single hair is about two to four years.
✓ Your genes determine how long a hair stays with you.
✓ If your hair is flat and lifeless try using a conditioner-free shampoo.
✓ Keep at least two to three different shampoos on-hand, switching them every week.
✓ Brushing your hair stimulates the scalp.
✓ Hair and nails are the only two places in the human body without red blood cells.
✓ Your diet can prevent hair loss!

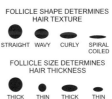

FOLLICLE SHAPE DETERMINES HAIR TEXTURE

STRAIGHT   WAVY   CURLY   SPIRAL COILED

FOLLICLE SIZE DETERMINES HAIR THICKNESS

THICK   THIN   THICK   THIN

Quick Tip 1: Purchasing shampoos that have added keratin, claiming to strengthen hair or promote hair growth, don't work. Protein rich foods do. They supply the nutrients needed to nourish the dermal papilla for hair growth.

Quick Tip 2: People who lack zinc and copper in their diets tend to have fine hair with less healthy follicles. A loss of strength to hold the hair shaft in place results in hair loss.

—— The Hairy Details ——

Below the surface of the skin is the hair root, which is enclosed within a hair follicle. At the base of the hair follicle is the dermal papilla. The dermal papilla is fed by the bloodstream which carries nourishment to produce new hair.

The Hair Growth Cycle:

The **Growth Phase** (Anagen phase) generally lasts about six to 10 years. At any one time, about 90% of hair is in the growth phase. How long this phase lasts is determined genetically, varies between the sexes and from one person to another.

The **Transitional Phase** (Catagen phase) is a very short, deactivation phase where the hair follicle prepares to go inactive; this lasts about two to three weeks.

The **Resting Phase** (Telogen phase) is the final phase of a hair follicle and lasts about 30 to 90 days. At any given time about 10% of the hair is in this phase. The hairs that come out when brushing are typically resting phase hair shafts.

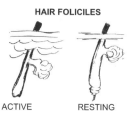

HAIR FOLICILES

ACTIVE   RESTING

Nail Facts at Your Fingertips

- ✓ Nails grow an average of two inches a year.
- ✓ Nail growth slows with age.
- ✓ Men's nails typically grow faster than women's (except during pregnancy or old age).
- ✓ Nails on the dominant hand tend to grow faster.
- ✓ The nails on your fingers grow faster than the nails on your toes.
- ✓ Drinking insufficient water can cause your nails to break.
- ✓ Ridges on your nail bed do not mean you have a serious medical condition.
- ✓ Wearing nail polish can help strengthen the nail (much like adding a coat of paint for protection).
- ✓ Applying lotions that contain alcohol can dry your nails, making them brittle.
- ✓ One in three Americans bites their fingernails.

Don't be surprised if at your next checkup your doctor takes a look at your nails. Even if you're having no problems with them, fingernails provide good clues to a person's overall health. For instance, when the doctor presses your nails, he or she is checking your blood circulation. By looking at your nails, a doctor may find changes that could be associated with skin problems, lung disease, anemia or other medical conditions.

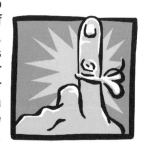

Scratching Below the Surface

Nails grow from the matrix (the root of the nail), the most important feature of the nail unit. This area is not visible; it is hidden and protected. The matrix produces keratin cells that make up the nail plate. The overall length of the matrix determines the thickness of the nail (the longer the matrix the thicker the nail). A short matrix produces fewer cells and a thinner nail. Matrix shapes and sizes vary by person. A flat matrix will produce a flat nail and a curved matrix will produce a curved nail. Damage to the matrix can cause permanent damage to the appearance of the nail.

The base of the fingernails and toenails (as well as along both sides of the nail) is embedded into the skin. Unlike other skin, this skin contains elastic fibers that connect it to the fingernail or toenail, holding them firmly in place. The cuticle, a rim of skin over the nail bed, protects it from bacterial infection, serves as a shock absorber and shields the nail from any sudden impacts.

Superfoods Shopping Chart

	Brain Power	Moods Stress	Heart Health	Weight Metabolism	Digestion Elimination	Immune	Joints Ligaments	Hair Nail Skin	Internal Cleansing
Adzuki Beans	√	√	√	√			√	√	
Aloe Vera Juice		√		√	√		√		√
Almonds	√	√		√			√	√	
Angostura Bitters			√	√	√				√
Apples			√	√	√	√		√	√
Artichoke			√	√	√	√			√
Asparagus			√	√			√	√	
Astragalus				√		√			
Avocado	√	√	√	√			√	√	√
Bananas		√			√				
Barley Grass	√	√	√	√	√	√	√	√	√
Barley-grain	√	√	√	√	√	√	√	√	
Bee Pollen	√		√	√		√			
Beets	√	√	√	√	√	√			√
Bitter Greens				√	√	√			√
Black Beans	√	√	√	√		√	√	√	
Blueberries	√		√	√		√		√	√
Bowellia							√		
Brazil Nuts	√	√	√	√	√	√	√	√	
Broccoli			√	√	√	√		√	√
Brown Rice	√	√	√	√	√		√		
Brussels Sprouts			√	√	√	√		√	√
Buckwheat	√	√	√	√			√	√	
Burdock Root				√	√	√			√
Cabbage		√		√	√	√		√	√
Cardamom Seeds				√	√				
Carrots	√	√	√	√			√	√	
Chickpeas	√	√	√	√			√	√	
Chicory			√	√	√	√			√
Chlorella	√		√	√	√	√		√	√
Chocolate	√	√	√	√					
Cinnamon		√	√	√	√		√		
Cranberries	√	√	√	√	√	√		√	√
Dandelion			√	√	√	√		√	√
Eggs, Enriched Omega-3	√	√	√	√			√	√	
Eleuthro	√	√		√		√			
Figs	√	√	√	√		√		√	√
Garlic			√	√		√			√
Ginger	√	√	√	√	√	√	√		√
Gingko Biloba	√	√	√						
Grape Juice, Purple	√	√	√	√		√		√	√
Grapefruit			√	√	√	√		√	√
Green Peas			√	√	√			√	√
Green Superfoods	√	√	√	√	√	√	√	√	√
Green Tea	√	√	√	√		√		√	√
Gruyere Cheese	√	√		√				√	√
Hops		√		√	√				
Horsetail Equisetum Avense	√					√	√	√	√
Jerusalem Artichoke	√	√		√	√	√			√
Kale			√	√	√	√	√	√	√
Kefir	√	√	√	√	√	√	√		√
Kimchi			√	√	√	√			√
Kiwi	√	√	√	√		√		√	√
Lecithin	√	√	√	√	√	√	√	√	√
Lemons				√	√	√	√	√	√
Lentil Beans	√	√	√	√		√	√	√	
Milk Thistle				√	√	√		√	√
Milk, Non Fat Dry	√	√	√	√			√	√	
Miso	√	√		√	√	√	√	√	
Mushrooms			√	√		√			
Mustard Greens	√	√	√	√	√		√	√	

175

Get Balanced – The Natural Way to Better Health with Superfoods

	Brain Power	Moods Stress	Heart Health	Weight Metabolism	Digestion Elimination	Immune	Joints Ligaments	Hair Nail Skin	Internal Cleansing
Nova Scotia Dulse				√		√		√	√
Nutritional Yeast	√	√	√	√	√	√	√	√	√
Oat Bran	√	√	√	√	√	√			√
Oatmeal	√	√	√	√	√	√			√
Olive Oil	√	√	√	√	√	√	√	√	√
Papaya				√	√	√		√	√
Parsley	√		√	√	√	√		√	√
Passion Flower		√		√	√				
Peppermint				√	√				√
Pineapple				√	√		√		√
Pistachio Nuts	√	√	√						
Pumpkin Seeds	√	√	√	√		√	√	√	
Quinoa	√	√	√	√	√		√	√	
Raspberries	√	√	√	√	√	√		√	√
Red Clover		√					√	√	√
Rosemary	√	√	√	√		√		√	√
Salmon	√	√	√	√		√	√	√	
Sardines	√	√	√	√		√	√	√	
Scallops	√	√	√	√		√	√	√	
Sea Vegetables	√	√	√	√	√	√	√	√	√
Shrimp	√	√	√	√				√	
Snapper	√	√	√	√		√	√	√	
Soybeans	√	√	√	√	√		√	√	
Spinach	√	√	√	√	√	√	√	√	√
Spirulina	√	√	√	√	√	√	√	√	√
St. John's Wort		√		√					
Steak, Lean Top Sirloin	√	√	√				√	√	
Strawberries	√	√	√	√	√	√		√	√
Sunflower Seeds	√	√	√	√			√	√	
Sweet Potato	√	√	√	√	√			√	
Swiss Chard	√	√	√	√	√		√	√	√
Tofu	√	√	√	√	√		√	√	
Tomato	√	√	√	√	√	√		√	√
Tuna	√	√	√	√		√	√	√	
Turmeric	√	√	√	√	√	√	√		
Turnip Greens	√	√	√	√	√	√	√	√	√
Valerian Root		√		√					
Walnuts	√	√	√	√		√		√	√
Watercress	√		√	√	√	√		√	√
Watermelon	√	√	√	√	√	√		√	√
Wheat Germ	√	√	√	√	√	√	√	√	√
Whey Powder	√	√	√	√			√	√	
Wild Rice	√	√	√	√	√	√		√	
Winter Squash	√	√	√	√	√	√		√	√
Yogurt	√	√	√	√	√	√	√	√	√

Resources and Notes

Chapter One – Superfoods for Brain Power

Joseph, J.A., et al. "Blueberry supplementation enhances signaling and prevents behavioral deficits in an Alzheimer disease model." *Nutr Neurosci.* 6(3):153-162, 2003.

Shukitt-Hale, B., et al. "Mechanisms involved in blueberry enhancements of motor and cognitive function in young and old rats." 33rd Annual Meeting of the Society for Neuroscience. New Orleans, USA. November 812, 2003.

Spangler, E.L., et al. "Rats fed a blueberry-enriched diet exhibit greater protection against a kainate-induced learning impairment." 33rd Annual Meeting of the Society for Neuroscience. New Orleans, USA. November 812, 2003.

Joseph, J.A., et al. "Reversals of age-related declines in neuronal signal transduction, cognitive, and motor behavioral deficits with blueberry, spinach, or strawberry dietary supplementation." *Journal of Neuroscience.* 19(18):8114-8121, 1999.

Goyarzu, P., et al. "Blueberry supplemented diet: effects on object recognition memory and nuclear factor-kappa B levels in aged rats." *Nutritional Neuroscience.* 7(2):75-83, 2004.

Goyarzu, P., et al. "Age-related increase in brain NF-kB is attenuated by blueberry-enriched antioxidant diet." 33rd Annual Meeting of the Society for Neuroscience. New Orleans, USA. November 812, 2003.

Safford, F., et al. "Testing the effects of dietary lecithin on memory in the elderly: An example of social work/medical research collaboration." *Research On Social Work Practice.* 4:349-358, 1994.

Dysken, M. "A review of recent clinical trials in the treatment of Alzheimer's disease." *Psychiatric Annals.* 17(3):178, 1987.

Little, A., et al. "A double-blind, placebo controlled trial of high-dose lecithin in Alzheimer's Disease." *Journal of Neurology, Neurosurgery and Psychiatry.* 48(8):736-742, 1985.

Volz, H.P., et al. "Improvement in quality of life in the elderly. Results of a placebo-controlled study on the efficacy and tolerability of lecithin fluid in patients with impaired cognitive functions." *MMW Fortschr Med.* 146:99-106, 2004.

Safford, F., et al. "Testing the effects of dietary lecithin on memory in the elderly: An example of social work/medical research collaboration." *Research On Social Work Practice.* 4:349-358, 1994.

Volz, H.P., et al. "Improvement in quality of life in the elderly. Results of a placebo-controlled study on the efficacy and tolerability of lecithin fluid in patients with impaired cognitive functions." *MMW Fortschr Med.* 146:99-106, 2004.

Dimpfel, W., et al. "Efficacy of dimethylaminoethanol (DMAE) containing vitamin-mineral drug combination on EEG patterns in the presence of different emotional states." *Eur J Med Res.* 8(5):183-191, 2003.

Murphree, H.B., et al. "The stimulant effect of 2-diethylaminoethanol (Deanol) in human volunteer subjects." *Clinical Pharmacology and Therapeutics.* 1:303-310, 1960.

Lewis, J.A., et al. "Deanol and methylphenidate in minimal brain dysfunction." *Clin Pharmacol Ther.* 17(5):534-540, 1975.

Engelhart, M.J., et al. "Dietary Intake of Antioxidants and Risk of Alzheimer Disease." *JAMA*. 287:3223-3229, 2002.

Zandi, P.P., et al. "Reduced risk of Alzheimer disease in users of antioxidant vitamin supplements." The Cache County Study. *Archives of Neurology*. 61:82-88, 2004.

Riviere, S., et al. "Low plasma vitamin C in Alzheimer patients despite an adequate diet." *Int J Geriatr Psychiatry*. 13(11):749-754, 1998.

Paleologos, M., et al. "Cohort study of vitamin C intake and cognitive impairment." *American Journal of Epidemiology*. 148(1):45-50, 1998.

Kubala, A.L., et al. "Nutritional factors in psychological test behavior." *Journal of Genetic Psychology*. 96:343-352, 1960.

Parle, M., et al. "Ascorbic acid: a promising memory-enhancer in mice." *J Pharmacol Sci*. 93(2):129-135, 2003.

Terpstra, M., et al. "1H NMR detection of vitamin C in human brain in vivo." *Magn Reson Med*. 51(2):225-229, 2004.

Sandyk R., Kanofsky, J.D., "Vitamin C in the treatment of schizophrenia." *Int J Neurosci*. 1993 Jan;68(1-2):67-71. Department of Psychiatry, Albert Einstein College of Medicine, Bronx, NY 10461. Entrez PubMed.

Russel T., et al. "Coenzyme Q10 administration increases brain mitochondrial concentration and exerts neuroprotective effects." *Proc Nat Acad Sci*. 1998;95:8892-7.

McDonald, S.R.; Sohal, R.S.; Forster, M.J.; "Concurrent administration of coenzyme Q10 and alpha-tocopherol improves learning in aged mice." Department of Pharmacology and Neuroscience, Institute for Aging and Alzheimer's Disease Research, University of North Texas Health Science Center at Fort Worth, Fort Worth, TX 76107, USA. Entrez PubMed INIST-CNRS, Cote INIST : 18809, 35400013497103.0040.

Cheng, J.P.; Hu, W.X.; Liu, X.J.; Zheng, M.; Shi, W.; Wang, W.H.; "Expression of c-fos and oxidative stress on brain of rats reared on food from mercury-selenium coexisting mining area." School of Environmental Science and Engineering, Shanghai Jiaotong University, China. jpcheng@sjtu.edu.cn. PMID: 15721983 [PubMed - indexed for MEDLINE].

Blount, B.C., et al. "Folate deficiency causes uracil misincorporation into human DNA and chromosome breakage: Implications for cancer and neuronal damage." *Proceedings of the National Academy of Sciences*, USA. 94:3290-3295, 1997.

Langlais, P.J., et al. "Thiamine deficiency in rats produces cognitive and memory deficits on spatial tasks that correlate with tissue loss in diencephalon, cortex and white matter." *Behav Brain Res*. 68(1):75-89, 1995.

Morris, M.C., et al. "Dietary niacin and the risk of incident Alzheimer's disease and of cognitive decline." *J Neuro Neurosurg Psychiatry*. 75:1093-1099, 2004.

Wei, I.L., et al. "Vitamin B(6) deficiency decreases the glucose utilization in cognitive brain structures of rats." *J Nutr Biochem*. 10(9):525-531, 1999.

Bryan, J., et al. "Associations between dietary intake of folate and vitamins B-12 and B-6 and self-reported cognitive function and psychological well-being in Australian men and women in midlife." *J Nutr Health Aging*. 8(4):226-232, 2004.CSIRO, Health Sciences and Nutrition, Adelaide, South Australia.

Morris, M.C., et al. "Consumption of fish and n-3 fatty acids and risk of incident Alzheimer disease." *Arch Neurol.* 60(7):940-946, 2003. Rush Institute for Healthy Aging, Department of Internal Medicine, Rush Alzheimer's Disease Center, Rush-Presbyterian St. Luke's Medical Center, Chicago, IL, USA.

Kidd, P.M. "Autism, an extreme challenge to integrative medicine. Part II: medical management." *Alternative Medicine Review.* 7(6):472-499, 2002. The B:W (Better:Worse with treatment) ratio reported by parents of autistic children for calcium is 14:1.

Haas (M.D.), Elson. "Calcium." Excerpted from *Staying Healthy with Nutrition: The Complete Guide to Diet and Nutritional Medicine,* Celestial Arts Books, 1992.

Youdim, M.B., et al. "Putative biological mechanisms of the effect of iron deficiency on brain biochemistry and behavior." *American Journal of Clinical Nutrition.* 50(3 Supplement):607-15, 1990.

Starobrat-Hermelin, B., et al. "The effects of magnesium physiological supplementation on hyperactivity in children with attention deficit hyperactivity disorder (ADHD). Positive response to magnesium oral loading test." *Magnes Res.* 10:149-156, 1997.

Kozielec, T., et al. "Assessment of magnesium levels in children with attention deficit hyperactivity disorder (ADHD)." *Magnesium Research.* 10(2):143-148, 1997.

Research at Washington University in St. Louis School of Medicine, by Lawrence Salkoff, Ph.D. Department of Anatomy & Neurobiology. Development, Function, and Regulation of Potassium Ion Channels.

Nowak, G., et al. "Mechanisms contributing to antidepressant zinc actions." *Pol J Pharmacol.* 54(6):587-592, 2002. Department of Neurobiology, Institute of Pharmacology, Polish Academy of Sciences, Krakow, Poland.

Penland, J.G. "Dietary boron, brain function, and cognitive performance." *Environ Health Perspect.* 102(Supplement 7):65-72, 1994.

Publication: Psyched for Success, Publication Date: 3 January 2003, Last Reviewed: 24 Jul 2006, (Document ID: 2517).

Fernstrom, J.D.; Fernstrom, M.H.; Grubb, P.E.; Volk, E.A.; "Absence of chronic effects of dietary protein content on brain tryptophan concentrations in rats." *J Nutr.* 1985 Oct;115(10):1337-44. PMID: 2413190 [PubMed - indexed for MEDLINE].

Chapter Two – Superfoods for Moods and Stress

Knopman, D., et al. "An open-label, 24-week pilot study of the methyl donor betaine in Alzheimer disease patients." *Alzheimer Dis Assoc Disord.* 15(3):162-165, 2001.

Kim, S.K., et al. "Effect of acute betaine administration on hepatic metabolism of S-amino acids in rats and mice." *Biochem Pharmacol.* 65(9):1565-1574, 2003.
College of Pharmacy, Seoul National University, Kwanak-Ku, Seoul, South Korea.

"Stephen Nottingham's meticulously researched online book, *Beetroot*" 2004, *The Times* (London), 15th August 2005 Nottingham, Stephen, 2003-2006. Science writer and journalist within project teams at ESN (European Service Network). Numerous research summaries, articles and reports for print and web publication.

Lee, K.W., et al. "Cocoa has more phenolic phytochemicals and a higher antioxidant capacity than teas and red wine." *J Agric Food Chem.* 51(25):7292-7295, 2003.

Drewnowski, A.; Krahn, D.D.; Demitrack, M.A.; Nairn, K.; Gosnell, B.A. "Taste responses and preferences for sweet high-fat foods: evidence for opioid involvement." *Physiol Behav.* 1992 Feb;51(2):371-9. Program in Human Nutrition, University of Michigan School of Public Health, Ann Arbor 48109-2029.

A Science odyssey, people and discoveries, role of endorphins discovered 1975, PBS.org

Dalayeun, J.F.; Nores, J.M.; Bergal, S. "Physiology of beta-endorphins. A close-up view and a review of the literature." *Biomed Pharmacother.* 1993;47(8):311-20. Hopital Suisse, issy-les-Moulineaux, France. PMID: 7520295 [PubMed - indexed for MEDLINE].

Krenn, L. "Passion Flower (Passiflora incarnata L.)--a reliable herbal sedative." *Wien Med Wochenschr.* 152(15-16):404-406, 2002.

Soulimani, R., et al. "Behavioural effects of Passiflora incarnata L. and its indole alkaloid and flavonoid derivatives and maltol in the mouse." *Journal of Ethnopharmacology.* 57(1):11-20, 1997.

Student Health Services, Oregon State University. Nutrition, Diet and Stress http://studenthealth.oregonstate.edu/topics/nutrition-diet-stress.php

Raloff, Janet. "Stress-prone? Altering the diet may help." Science News Online, March 10, 2001, vol 159, no 10.

Akhondzadeh, S.; Naghavi, H.R.; Vazirian, M.; Shayeganpour, A.; Rashidi, H.; Khani, M. "Passionflower in the treatment of generalized anxiety: a pilot double-blind randomized controlled trial with oxazepam." *J Clin Pharm Ther.* 2001 Oct;26(5):363-7. Roozbeh Psychiatric Hospital, Tehran University of Medical Sciences, South Kargar Avenue, Tehran, Iran. s.akhond@neda.net

Bottiglieri, T., et al. "The clinical potential of ademetionine (S-adenosylmethionine) in neurological disorders." *Drugs.* 48(2):137-152, 1994.

Ngueyn, T.T., et al. "Effect of vitamin B6 deficiency on the synthesis and accumulation of S-adenosylhomocysteine and S-adenosylmethionine in rat tissues." *J Nutr Sci Vitaminol.* 47(3):188-194, 2001.

Verdon, F., et al. "Iron supplementation for unexplained fatigue in non-anaemic women: double blind randomised placebo controlled trial." *BMJ.* 326(7399):1124, 2003. General Practice Unit, University of Lausanne, Lausanne, Switzerland.

Better Health, Health and Medical information for consumers, quality assured by the Victorian government (Australia), Iron Explained. www.betterhealth.vic.gov

Zieba, A., et al. "Serum trace elements in animal models and human depression: Part III. Magnesium. Relationship with copper." *Hum Psychopharmacol.* 15(8):631-635, 2000. Department of Psychiatry, Collegium Medicum, Jagiellonian University, Krakow, Poland.

Cernak, I., et al. "Alterations in magnesium and oxidative status during chronic emotional stress." *Magnesium Research.* 13(1):29-36, 2000.

Johnson, S., et al. "The multifaceted and widespread pathology of magnesium deficiency." *Medical Hypotheses.* 56(2):163-170, 2001.Excessive stress causes the depletion of magnesium.

Kaemmerer, K., et al. "Studies on magnesium. 3. Effect of magnesium aspartate hydrochloride on stress reactions in magnesium-deficient animals." *Zentralbl Veterinarmed A.* 31(5):334-339, 1984

Hass, op. cit. Minerals Magnesium, pp.170-71.

Briggs, S. "Magnesiuma forgotten mineral." *Health & Nutrition Breakthroughs.* November 1997.

Nowak, G., et al. "Effect of zinc supplementation on antidepressant therapy in unipolar depression: a preliminary placebo-controlled study." *Pol J Pharmacol.* 55(6):1143-1147, 2003. Department of Neurobiology, Institute of Pharmacology, Polish Academy of Sciences, Poland.

Cox, J. R., et al. "Changes in sodium, potassium and fluid spaces in depression and dementia." *Gerontology Clin.* 13:232-245, 1971.

Webb, W. L., et al. "Electrolyte and fluid imbalance: Neuropsychiatric manifestations." *Psychosomatics.* 22(3):199-203, 1981.

Marano, Hara Estroff. "An A for Vitamin C. Vitamin C doesn't just fight coldsit can lower stress too!" *Psychology Today Magazine*, October 2, 2002,(Document ID: 2303)

Hass, op. cit. Vitamin A and Vitamin C, p. 97.

Adams, P. B., et al. "Arachidonic acid to eicosapentaenoic acid ratio in blood correlates positively with clinical symptoms of depression." *Lipids.* 31(Supplement):S157-S161, 1996.

Frasure-Smith, N., et al. "Major depression is associated with lower omega-3 fatty acid levels in patients with recent acute coronary syndromes." *Biol Psychiatry.* 55(9):891-896, 2004.

Chapter Three – Superfoods for Internal Cleansing

Kuoroda, T., et al. "Bile acids in hepatic bile in liver disease." *Acta Hepato Gastroenterol.* 21:120-126, 1974.

Gebhardt, R. "Antioxidative and protective properties of extracts from leaves of the artichoke (Cynara scolymus L.) against hydroperoxide-induced oxidative stress in cultured rat hepatocytes." *Toxicol Appl Pharmacol.* 144(2):279-286, 1997.

Nooroozi, M., et al. "Effects of flavonoids and vitamin C on oxidative DNA damage to human lymphocytes." *American Journal of Clinical Nutrition.* 67(6):1210-1218, 1998.

"Stephen Nottingham's meticulously researched online book, *Beetroot*" 2004, *The Times* (London), 15th August 2005 Nottingham, Stephen, 2003-2006. Science writer and journalist within project teams at ESN (European Service Network). Numerous research summaries, articles and reports for print and web publication.

Walters, D. G., et al. "Cruciferous vegetable consumption alters the metabolism of the dietary carcinogen 2-amino-1-methyl-6-phenylimidazo[4,5-b]pyridine (PhIP) in humans." *Carcinogenesis.* 2004.

Hass, op. cit. Wheat grass and Barley grass, p. 282.

Fitzgerald, Dr. Patricia. *The Detox Solution, the Missing Link to Radiant Health, Abundant Energy, Ideal Weight, and Peace of Mind.* (Illumination Press, 2001.); p. 274, chlorophyll.

Berry, Linda (D.C.). *Internal Cleansing.* (Three Rivers Press, NY, 2000).

Pedersen, Mark. *Nutritional Herbology, a Reference Guide to Herbs.* (Wendell W. Whitman Company, 2002)

Sobota, A. E., et al. "Inhibition of bacterial adherence by cranberry juice: potential for use for the treatment of urinary tract infections." *Journal of Urology.* 31:1013-1016, 1984.

Kontiokari, T., et al. "Randomised trial of cranberry-lingonberry juice and Lactobacillus GG drink for the prevention of urinary tract infections in women." *British Medical Journal.* 322(7302):1571, 2001.

Ofek, I.; Goldhar, J.; Zafriri, D.; Lis, H.; Adar, R.; Sharon, N. "Anti-Escherichia coli adhesion activity of cranberry and blueberry juices." *New England Journal of Medicine* 1991; 324: 1599.

Howell, A.B.; Reed, J.; Winterbottom, R.; Krueger, C. "Bacterial anti-adhesion activity of cranberry vs. other foods." *Federation of American Societies for Experimental Biology Journal* 2002.

Howell, A.B.; Leahy, M.; Kurowska, E.; Guthrie, N. "In vivo evidence that cranberry proanthocyanidins inhibit adherence of p-fimbriated E. coli bacteria to uroepithelial cells." *Federation of American Societies for Experimental Biology Journal* 2001; 15: A284.

US National Library of Medicine and the National Institute of Health, Medline Plus, Dandelion (taraxacum officinale), updated December 13, 2005.

Fitzgerald, op. cit. p. 267, limonene.

Haas, op. cit.; p. 301, Lemons and Grapefruits.

Schechter, Steven R., N.D. *Fighting Radiation & Chemicals Pollutants with Foods, Herbs and Vitamins.* (Vitality Ink Books, 1988), p. 72, Sea Vegetables; p. 61, boosting your immunity with Vitamin A.

Fitzgerald, op. cit.; p. 295, milk thistle; p. 248, vitamins for detoxing; pp. 263-70, Phytonutrients.

Magliulo, E., et al. "Results of a double blind study on the effect of silymarin in the treatment of acute viral hepatitis, carried out at two medical centres." *Med Klin.* 73:1060-1065, 1978

Pietrangelo, A., et al. "Iron-induced oxidant stress in nonparenchymal liver cells: mitochondrial derangement and fibrosis in acutely iron-dosed gerbils and its prevention by silybin." *J Bioenerg Biomembr.* 34(1):67-79, 2002.

Kreeman, V., et al. "Silymarin inhibits the development of diet-induced hypercholesterolemia in rats." *Planta Medica.* 64:138-142, 1998.

Nassuato, G., et al. "Effect of silibinin on biliary lipid composition: experimental and clinical study. *J Hepatol.*" 12:290-295, 1991.

Thiamin may have antioxidant, erythropoietic, cognition-and mood-modulatory, antiatherosclerotic and detoxification activities. It has putative ergogenic activity. Thiamin has been found to protect against lead-induced lipid peroxidation in rat liver and kidney http://www.pdrhealth.com/drug_info/nmdrugprofiles/nutsupdrugs/thi_0261.shtml

Murray, Michael T. (ND) *Encyclopedia of Nutritional Supplements.* Prima Publishing, 1996.

List of phytochemicals and their breakdowns:
http://www.phytochemicals.info/phytochemicals.php

Glossary and Pronunciation of Functional Food Terms
http://www.arfunctionalfoods.org/Consumer/glossary_definitions.htm

Norman, Helen; Go, Vay Liang W.; Butrum, Ritva R. *Journal of Nutrition*, December 2004, International Research Conference on food, Nutrition, and Cancer.

Chapter Four – Superfoods for Digestion and Elimination

Langmead, L., et al. "Anti-inflammatory effects of aloe vera gel in human colorectal mucosa in vitro." *Aliment Pharmacol Ther.* 19(5):521-527, 2004.

Centre for Adult and Paediatric Gastroenterology, Institute of Cellular and Molecular Science, Barts and the London, Queen Mary School of Medicine and Dentistry, London, UK.

Robinson, M. "Medical therapy of inflammatory bowel disease for the 21st century." *European Journal of Surgery.* Supplement: 582, 1998. The author indicates that acemannan derived from Aloe vera is emerging as a promising treatment for inflammatory bowel disease.

Roberts, A. J., et al. *Nutraceuticals: the Complete Encyclopedia of Supplements, Herbs, Vitamins and Healing Foods.* Berkely Publishing Group. New York, USA. 2001:93.

Brewer, Dr. Sarah. *Good Digestion Guide*, July 2004. Healthspan.co.uk
Aloe vera has a soothing effect on bowel function. It normalizes bowel contraction, improves protein digestion and absorption, aids stool bulk and promotes a healthy balance of bowel bacteria.

Eamlamnam, K.; Patumraj, S.; Visedopas, N.; Thong-Ngam, D. "Effects of Aloe vera and sucralfate on gastric microcirculatory changes, cytokine levels and gastric ulcer healing in rats." *World J Gastroenterol.* 2006 Apr 7;12(13):2034-9. Department of Physiology, Faculty of Medicine, Chulalongkorn University, Bangkok 10330, Thailand.

Bartram, Thomas. *Bartram's Encyclopedia of Herbal Medicine.* Grace Publishers, 1995. Gentian, p. 197; dandelion, p. 140; papaya, p. 327; parsley, p. 329; peppermint, p. 331.

Pannangpetch, P., et al. "The antiulcerative effect of Thai Musa species in rats." *Phytotherapy Research.* 15(5):407-410, 2001. Departments of Pharmacology, Pathology and Parasitology, Faculty of Medicine, Khon Kaen University, Khon Kaen, Thailand.

Alberta Government, Agricultural, Food and Rural Development Dr. Thava Vasanthan, Associate Professor, Grain Science and Technology Department of Agricultural, Food and Nutritional Science, University of Alberta, Edmonton, Alberta, Canada Presented at the 3rd Canadian Barley Symposium, June 19-20, 2003.

Murray, N.D., Michael; Pizzorno, N.D., Joseph; Pizzorno, M.A., Lara. *The Encyclopedia of Healing Foods.* Atria Books 2005. Dandelion, pp. 109-91; arugula, pp. 160-61; chicory, pp. 196-97.

Cheney, G. "Rapid healing of peptic ulcers in patients receiving fresh cabbage juice." *Cal Med.* 1949;70:10.

Doll, R.; Pygott, F. "Clinical trial of Robaden and of cabbage juice in the treatment of gastric ulcer." *Lancet.* 1954;2:1200.

Thaly, H. "A new therapy of peptic ulcer: The anti-ulcer factor of cabbage." *Gaz Med Fr* 1965;72:1992-3.

Wikipedia, the free encyclopedia, Cardamon http://en.wikipedia.org/wiki/Cardamom

Willetts, K.E., et al. "Effect of a ginger extract on pregnancy-induced nausea: a randomised controlled trial." *Aust N Z J Obstet Gynaecol.* 43(2):139-144, 2003.
School of Women and Children's Health, University of New South Wales, Royal Hospital for Women, Randwick, New South Wales, Australia.

Pace, J.C. "Oral ingestion of encapsulated ginger and reported self care actions for the relief of chemotherapy-associated nausea and vomiting." *Dissertaion Abstr Internat.* 8:3297, 1987.

Lagarrigue, J.; Lazorthes, Y.; Verdie. J.C.; Richaud, J. "Analysis of the results of surgery and nucleolysis using papain in 1085 cases of lumbar disk hernias." *Neurochirurgie.* 1991;37(2):96-104; discussion 104-5. Service de Neurochirurgie, C.H.U. Toulouse Rangueil.

Zucker, S.; Buttle, D.J.; Nicklin, M.J.; Barrett, A.J. "The proteolytic activities of chymopapain, papain, and papaya proteinase III." *Biochim Biophys Acta.* 985 Apr 5;828(2):196-204. PMID: 3919769 PubMed - indexed for MEDLINE.

Kreydiyyeh, S.I., et al. "Diuretic effect and mechanism of action of parsley." *Journal of Ethnopharmacology.* 79(3):353-357, 2002.

May, B., et al. "Efficacy of a fixed peppermint/caraway oil combination in non-ulcer dyspepsia." *Arzneimittelforschung.* 46(12):1149-1153, 1996.

Liu, J.H., et al. "Enteric-coated peppermint-oil capsules in the treatment of irritable bowel syndrome: a prospective, randomized trial." *J Gastroenterol.* 32(6):765-768, 1997.

Health Encyclopedia, http://healthlibrary.epnet.com. "What Is the Scientific Evidence for Peppermint?" Pittler, M.H.; Ernst E. "Peppermint oil for irritable bowel syndrome: a critical review and meta-analysis." *Am J Gastroenterol.* 1998;93:1131-1135. Grigoleit, H.G.; Grigoleit, P. "Peppermint oil in irritable bowel syndrome." *Phytomedicine.* 2005;12:601-6.

Health Encyclopedia, http://healthlibrary.epnet.com. "What Is the Scientific Evidence for Bromelain?" Taussig, S.J,; Yokoyama, M.M.; Chinen, A., et al. "Bromelain, a proteolytic enzyme and its clinical application. A review." *Hiroshima J Med Sci.* 1975;24:185-193.
Taussig, S.J.; Batkin, S. "Bromelain, the enzyme complex of pineapple (Ananas comosus) and its clinical application. An update." *J Ethnopharmacol.* 1988;22:191-203.

Health Encyclopedia, http://healthlibrary.epnet.com. "What Is Turmeric Used for Today?" Deodhar, S.D.; Sethi, R.; Srimal, R.C. "Preliminary study on antirheumatic activity of curcumin (diferuloyl methane)." *Indian J Med Res.* 1980;71:632634. Ruby, A.J.; Kuttan, G.; Babu, K.D., et al. "Anti-tumour and antioxidant activity of natural curcuminoids." *Cancer Lett.* 1995;79-83. Satoskar, R.R.; Shah, S.J.; Shenoy, S.G. "Evaluation of anti-inflammatory property of curcumin (diferuloyl methane) in patients with postoperative inflammation." *Int J Clin Pharmacol Ther Toxicol.* 1986 Dec;24(12):651-654.

McCullough, F.S., et al. "The effect of vitamin A on epithelial integrity. *Proc Nutr Soc.* 58(2):289-293, 1999. Northern Ireland Centre for Diet and Health (NICHE), University of Ulster, Coleraine, UK.

Kozakova, H., et al. "Vitamin A deficiency leads to severe functional disturbance of the intestinal epithelium enzymes associated with diarrhoea and increased bacterial translocation in gnotobiotic rats." *Microbes Infect.* 5(5):405-411, 2003. Department of Immunology and Gnotobiology, Institute of Microbiology, Academy of Sciences of the Czech Republic, Novy Hradek, Czech Republic.

Prousky, J.E., et al. "Niacin (nicotinic acid) a putative treatment for hypochlorhydria: re-analysis of two case reports." *Journal of Orthomolecular Medicine.* 17(3):163-170, 2002.

Prousky, J.E. "Is vitamin B3 dependency a causal factor in the development of hypochlorhydria and achlorhydria?" *Journal of Orthomolecular Medicine.* 16(4): 225-237, 2001. Canadian College of Naturopathic Medicine.

Kelly, G.S., et al. "Pantethine: a review of its biochemistry and therapeutic applications." *Alternative Medicine Review.* 2(5):365-377, 1997.

Sachs, M., et al. "The metabolism of panthenol in patients with postoperative intestinal atony." *Z Ernahrungswiss.* 9(4):270-283, 1990.

Ely, J.T. "Aneurysm: prevention and nonsurgical repair." *Med Sci Monit.* 10(1):HY1-4, 2004.

Sasazuki, S., et al. "The effect of 5-year vitamin C supplementation on serum pepsinogen level and Helicobacter pylori infection." *Cancer Sci.* 94(4):378-382, 2003. Epidemiology and Biostatistics Division, National Cancer Center Research Institute East, Kashiwa, Japan.

Ozdil, S., et al. "Protective effects of ascorbic acid, dl-a-tocopherol acetate, and sodium selenate on ethanol-induced gastric mucosal injury of rats." *Biol Trace Elem Res.* 99(1-3):173-190, 2004. Department of Internal Medicine, Istanbul Medical Faculty, Istanbul University, Turkey.

D'Odorico, A., et al. "Reduced plasma antioxidant concentrations and increased oxidative DNA damage in inflammatory bowel disease." *Scand J Gastroenterol.* 36(12):1289-1294, 2001.

Ademoglu, E., et al. "Do vitamin E and selenium have beneficial effects on trinitrobenzenesulfonic acid-induced experimental colitis?" *Dig Dis Sci.* 49(1):102-108, 2004. Department of Biochemistry, Istanbul Faculty of Medicine, Istanbul University, Istanbul, Turkey.

Semba, R.D., et al. "Carotenoid and vitamin E status are associated with indicators of sarcopenia among older women living in the community." *Aging Clin Exp Res.* 15(6):482-487, 2003. The Johns Hopkins Medical Institutions, Baltimore, MD, USA.

Brzozowski, T., et al. "Role of L-arginine, a substrate for nitric oxide-synthase, in gastroprotection and ulcer healing." Journal of Gastroenterology. 32(4):442-452, 1997. Institute of Physiology and Pathophysiology, Jagiellonian University of Medicine, Krakow, Poland.

Brzozowski, T., et al. "Healing of chronic gastric ulcerations by L-arginine. Role of nitric oxide, prostaglandins, gastrin and polyamines." *Digestion.* 56(6):463-471, 1995. Institute of Physiology, Jagiellonian University School of Medicine, Krakow, Poland.

Watanabe, G., et al. "Effects of oral administration of L-arginine on renal function in patients with heart failure." *J Hypertens.* 18(2):229-234, 2000.

Schneider, R., et al. "l-Arginine counteracts nitric oxide deficiency and improves the recovery phase of ischemic acute renal failure in rats." *Kidney Int.* 64(1):216-225, 2003. Division of Nephrology, Department of Medicine, Julius-Maximilians-University, Wurzburg, Germany; andRudolf-Buchheim-Institute for Pharmacology, Justus-Liebig-University, Giessen, Germany.

Fallon, Sally; Enig, Mary G. (PhD.). *The Long Hollow Tube: A Primer on the Digestive System.*

The Weston A. Price Foundation, PMB 106-380, 4200 Wisconsin Ave., NW, Washington DC 20016.

Barbarino, F., et al. "Effects of zinc-aspartate and zinc-glycinate in healthy rats and on reserpine-induced gastric lesions." *Biol Trace Elem Res.* 16(3):253-267, 1988.

Daniele, B., et al. "Oral glutamine in the prevention of fluorouracil induced intestinal toxicity: a double blind, placebo controlled, randomised trial." *Gut.* 48:28-33, 2001.

Chen, G., et al. "Clinical observation of the protective effect of oral feeding of glutamine granules on intestinal mucous membrane." *Zhonghua Shao Shang Za Zhi.* 17(4):210-211, 2001.

Swarm, R.A., et al. "Protective effect of exogenous phospholipid on aspirin-induced gastric mucosal injury." *Am J Surgery.* 53(1):48-53, 1987.

Leyck, S., et al. "Improvement of the gastric tolerance of non-steroidal anti-inflammatory drugs by polyene phosphatidylcholine (Phospholipon 100)." *Eur J Pharmacol.* 17(1):35-42, 1985.

Chapter Five – Superfoods for Heart Health

Franziska, M.T., et al. "Effect of methionine loading on 5-methyltetrahydrofolate, S-adenosylmethionine and S-adenosylhomocysteine in plasma of healthy humans." *Clinical Science.* 91:79-86, 1996.

McCue, Kevin. "Cranberry Juice and Good Cholesterol." Chemistry.org, March 31, 2003. Raloff, Janet. Science News Online, March 29, 2003 Vol.163, No 13.

Lau, B.H.S., et al. "Allium sativum (garlic) and atherosclerosis: A review." *Nutrition Research.* 3:119-128, 1983.

Orekhov, A.N., et al. "Direct anti-atherosclerosis-related effects of garlic." *Ann Med.* 27(1):63-65, 1995.

Breithaupt-Grogler, K., et al. "Protective effect of chronic garlic intake on elastic properties of aorta in the elderly." *Circulation.* 96(8):2649-2655, 1997.

Tattelman, Dr. Ellen. "Health Effects of Garlic." *American Family Physician*, July 1, 2005. Albert Einstein College of Medicine of Yeshiva University, Bronx, New York.

Budoff, M.J.; Takasu, J.; Flores, F.R.; Niihara, Y.; Lu, B.; Lau, B.H.; Rosen, R.T.; Amagase, H. "Inhibiting progression of coronary calcification using Aged Garlic Extract in patients receiving statin therapy: a preliminary study." *Prev Med.* 2004 Nov;39(5):985-91. Division of Cardiology, Harbor-UCLA Medical Center Research and Education Institute, Torrance, CA 90502, USA. Budoff@Flash.net

Gorinstein, S.; Caspi, A.; Libman, I.; Lerner, H.T.; Huang, D.; Leontowicz. H.; Leontowicz, M.; Tashma, Z.; Katrich, E.; Feng, S.; Trakhtenberg, S. "Red grapefruit positively influences serum triglyceride level in patients suffering from coronary atherosclerosis: studies in vitro and in humans." *J Agric Food Chem.* 2006 Mar 8;54(5):1887-92. Department of Medicinal Chemistry and Natural Products, School of Pharmacy, The Hebrew University-Hadassah Medical School, P.O. Box 12065, Jerusalem 91120, Israel. gorin@cc.huji.ac.il

Won, S.M.; Park, Y.H.; Kim, H.J.; Park, K.M.; Lee, W.J. "Catechins inhibit angiotensin II-induced vascular smooth muscle cell proliferation via mitogen-activated protein kinase pathway." *Exp Mol Med.* 2006 Oct 31;38(5):525-34. Department of Physiology, School of Medicine, Kyungpook National University, Daegu 700-422, Korea.

Lin, J.K.; Lin-Shiau, S.Y. "Mechanisms of hypolipidemic and anti-obesity effects of tea and tea polyphenols." *Mol Nutr Food Res.* 2006 Feb;50(2):211-7. Institute of Pharmacology, College of Medicine, National Taiwan University, Taipei, Taiwan. jklin@ha.mc.ntu.edu.tw

Van Horn, Linda; Ph.D, RD for the Nutrition Committee. "Fiber, Lipids, and Coronary Heart Disease" Year Published: 1997 Product Code: 71-0113. A Statement for Healthcare Professionals From the Nutrition Committee, American Heart Association. 1997;95:2701-2704.

PC Oat Beta Glucan (Schiff), NSC-24 Immune Enhancer (Nutritional Supply Corp.), Maitake Bio-Beta-Glucan (Nature's Answer).

Biorklund, M.; van Rees, A.; Mensink, R.P.; Onning, G. "Changes in serum lipids and postprandial glucose and insulin concentrations after consumption of beverages with beta-glucans from oats or barley: a randomised dose-controlled trial." *Eur J Clin Nutr.* 2005 Nov;59(11):1272-81. Biomedical Nutrition, Center for Chemistry and Chemical Engineering, Lund University, Lund, Sweden.

Covas, M.I.; Nyyssonen, K.; Poulsen, H.E.; Kaikkonen, J.; Zunft, H.J.; Kiesewetter, H.; Gaddi, A.; de la Torre, R.; Mursu, J.; Baumler, H.; Nascetti, S.; Salonen, J.T.; Fito, M.; Virtanen, J.; Marrugat, J. "The effect of polyphenols in olive oil on heart disease risk factors: a randomized trial." *Ann Intern Med. 2006 Sep 5;145(5):153.*EUROLIVE Study Group. Municipal Institute for Medical Research, Barcelona, Spain. mcovas@imim.es

Med Health R I. 2006 Mar;89(3):113. "Olive oil in the treatment of hypercholesterolemia." Cullinen K. Rhode Island Comprehensive Cancer Control Program, Rhode Island Department of Health, USA.

Alonso, A.; Ruiz-Gutierrez, V.; Martinez-Gonzalez, M.A. "Monounsaturated fatty acids, olive oil and blood pressure: epidemiological, clinical and experimental evidence." *Public Health Nutr.* 2006 Apr;9(2):251-7. Department of Preventive Medicine and Public Health, School of Medicine, University of Navarra, Irunlarrea 1, ES-31008 Pamplona, Spain.

Rodriguez-Rodriguez, R.; Perona, J.S.; Herrera, M.D.; Ruiz-Gutierrez, V. "Triterpenic compounds from "orujo" olive oil elicit vasorelaxation in aorta from spontaneously hypertensive rats." *J Agric Food Chem.* 2006 Mar 22;54(6):2096-102. Instituto de la Grasa (CSIC), Avenida Padre Garcia Tejero 4, 41012 Seville, Spain.

Perona, J.S.; Canizares, J.; Montero, E.; Sanchez-Dominguez, J.M.; Catala, A.; Ruiz-Gutierrez, V. "Virgin olive oil reduces blood pressure in hypertensive elderly subjects." *Clin Nutr.* 2004 Oct;23(5):1113-21. Instituto de la Grasa, Consejo Superior de Investigaciones Cientificas, Avda. Padre Garcia Tejero 4, Sevilla 41012, Spain.

Connor, W.E.; Lin, D.S.; Pappu, A.S.; Frohlich, J.; Gerhard, G. "Dietary sitostanol and campestanol: accumulation in the blood of humans with sitosterolemia and xanthomatosis and in rat tissues." *Lipids.* 2005 Sep;40(9):919-23. Division of Endocrinology, Diabetes and Clinical Nutrition, Department of Medicine, L465, Oregon Health & Science University, Portland 97239-3098, USA. connorw@ohsu.edu

Pharmacol Res. 1999 Sep;40(3):211-25. Comment in: Pharmacol Res. 1999 Sep;40(3):203. Pharmacol Res. 1999 Sep;40(3):205-6. Health benefits of docosahexaenoic acid (DHA)Horrocks LA, Yeo YK. Docosa Foods Ltd, 1275 Kinnear Road, Columbus, OH 43212-1155, USA.

American Heart Assoc., July 2004 article: "Eating Broiled, Baked Fish May Lower Incidence Of Irregular Heart Rhythm In The Elderly." Cited Harvard Study.

Circulation. 2004 Jul 27;110(4):368-73. Epub 2004 Jul 19. Comment in: *Circulation.* 2005 Feb 1;111(4):e37; author reply e37. "Fish intake and risk of incident atrial fibrillation." Mozaffarian, D.; Psaty, B.M.; Rimm, E.B.; Lemaitre, R.N.; Burke, G.L.; Lyles, M.F.; Lefkowitz, D.; Siscovick, D.S. Channing Laboratory, Brigham and Women's Hospital and Harvard Medical School, and Department of Epidemiology, Harvard School of Public Health, Boston, Mass, USA. darymd@hotmail.com

Seierstad, S.L.; Seljeflot, I.; Johansen, O.; Hansen, R.; Haugen, M.; Rosenlund, G.; Froyland, L.; Arnesen, H. "Dietary intake of differently fed salmon; the influence on markers of human atherosclerosis." *Eur J Clin Invest.* 2005 Jan;35(1):52-9. The Norwegian School of Veterinary Science, Oslo, Norway.

Harvard School of Public Health, Oct. 2006, New study shows the benefits of eating fish greatly outweigh the risks. *Fish Consumption Associated With Reduced Risk of Cardiac Death, Lower Total Mortality, and Improvements in Child Brain Development.*

NutritionData.com, sunflower seeds, scallops. NutritionData (ND) provides a complete nutrient analysis for any food or recipe, and helps you select foods that best match your dietary needs.

Chapidze, G.E.; Kapanadze, S.D.; Dolidze, N.K.; Latsabidze, N.E.; Bakhutashvili, Z.V. "Combination treatment with coenzyme Q10 and simvastatin in patients with coronary atherosclerosis." *Kardiologiia.* 2006;46(8):11-3.

Sander, S.; Coleman, C.I.; Patel, A.A.; Kluger, J.; White, C.M. "The impact of coenzyme Q10 on systolic function in patients with chronic heart failure." *J Card Fail.* 2006 Aug;12(6):464-72. University of Connecticut School of Pharmacy, Storrs, Connecticut 06269, USA.

Tuekpe, M.K.; Todoriki, H.; Sasaki, S.; Zheng, K.C.; Ariizumi, M. "Potassium excretion in healthy Japanese women was increased by a dietary intervention utilizing home-parcel delivery of Okinawan vegetables." *Hypertens Res.* 2006 Jun;29(6):389-96. Department of Environmental and Preventive Medicine, Faculty of Medicine, University of the Ryukyus, Nishihara-cho, Okinawa, Japan.

Flight, I.; Clifton, P. "Cereal grains and legumes in the prevention of coronary heart disease and stroke: a review of the literature." *Eur J Clin Nutr.* 2006 Oct;60(10):1145-59. Epub 2006 May 3. CSIRO Human Nutrition, Adelaide, South Australia, Australia.

Inoue, I. "Lipid metabolism and magnesium." *Clin Calcium.* 2005 Nov;15(11):65-76. Department of Endocrinology and Diabetes, Saitama Medical School.

Song, Y.; Manson, J.E.; Cook, N.R.; Albert, C.M.; Buring, J.E.; Liu, S. "Dietary magnesium intake and risk of cardiovascular disease among women." *Am J Cardiol.* 2006 Jul 1;98(1):140.
Division of Preventive Medicine, Department of Medicine, Brigham and Women's Hospital, Harvard Medical School, Boston, Massachusetts, USA.

Lindeman, R.D.; Romero, L.J.; Yau, C.L.; Koehler, K.M.; Baumgartner, R.N.; Garry, P.J. "Serum homocysteine concentrations and their relation to serum folate and vitamin B12 concentrations and coronary artery disease prevalence in an urban, bi-ethnic community." *Ethn Dis.* 2003 Spring;13(2):178-85. Department of Internal Medicine, University of New Mexico School of Medicine, Albuquerque, New Mexico 87131-5666, USA.

Ito, Y.; Kurata, M.; Suzuki, K.; Hamajima, N.; Hishida, H.; Aoki, K. "Cardiovascular disease mortality and serum carotenoid levels: a Japanese population-based follow-up study." *J Epidemiol.* 2006 Jul;16(4):154-60. Department of Preventive Medicine/Biostatistics and Medical Decision Making, Nagoya University Graduate School of Medicine, Japan.

Hou, J.W. "Primary systemic carnitine deficiency presenting as recurrent Reye-like syndrome and dilated cardiomyopathy." *Chang Gung Med J.* 2002 Dec;25(12):832-7. Division of Medical Genetics, Department of Pediatrics, Chang Gung Children's Hospital, Taoyuan, Taiwan, ROC.

Böhmer, Thomas; Rydning, Andreas; Solberg, Helge Erik. "Carnitine levels in human serum in health and disease." Department of Medicine B, and Institute of Clinical Biochemistry, Rikshospitalet, University of Oslo, Oslo, Norway. Received 11 June 1974. Available online 15 January 2003.

Lourenco, R.; Camilo, M.E. "Taurine: a conditionally essential amino acid in humans? An overview in health and disease." *Nutr Hosp.* 2002 Nov-Dec;17(6):262-70. Servicos Farmaceuticos do Hospital de Santa Maria, Lisbon, Portugal.

American Heart Association Nutrition Committee. "Diet and lifestyle recommendations revision 2006: a scientific statement from the American Heart Association Nutrition Committee." *Circulation.* 2006 Jul 4;114(1):82-96. Epub 2006 Jun 19.

Circulation. 2003;107:e2.) © 2003 American Heart Association, Inc. "Exercise and Cardiovascular Health," Jonathan Myers, PhD From the Cardiology Division, VA Palo Alto Health Care System, Stanford University, Palo Alto, Calif. Correspondence to Jonathan Myers, PhD, Cardiology 111-C, VA Palo Alto Health Care System, 3801 Miranda Ave, Palo Alto, CA 94304.

Roizen, Dr. Michael F.; Oz, Dr. Mehmet C. *You the Owner's Manual.* Harper Resource books, 2005.

Chapter Six – Superfoods for Immune System

Nelson, Nancy. "The Majority of Cancers Are Linked to the Environment." National Cancer Institute, US National Institues of Health. June 17, 2004.

Brush, J.; Mendenhall, E.; Guggenheim, A.; Chan, T.; Connelly, E.; Soumyanath, A.; Buresh, R.; Barrett, R.; Zwickey, H. "The effect of Echinacea purpurea, Astragalus membranaceus and Glycyrrhiza glabra on CD69 expression and immune cell activation in humans." *Phytother Res.* 2006 Aug;20(8):687-95. Helfgott Research Institute, National College of Naturopathic Medicine, Portland, OR, USA.

Shao, B.M.; Xu, W.; Dai, H.; Tu, P.; Li, Z.; Gao, X.M. "A study on the immune receptors for polysaccharides from the roots of Astragalus membranaceus, a Chinese medicinal herb." *Biochem Biophys Res Commun.* 2004 Aug 6;320(4):1103-11. Department of Immunology, School of Basic Medical Science, Peking University Health Science Center, Beijing, China.

Block, K.I., Mead, M.N. "Immune system effects of echinacea, ginseng, and astragalus: a review." *Integr Cancer Ther.* 2003 Sep;2(3):247-67. Institute for Integrative Cancer Care and Block Center for Integrative Cancer Care, Evanston, Illinois 60201, USA. research@blockmedical.com

Medical News Today, 21 Aug 2006: "Three Common Herbs Effective In Boosting Key Lymphocytes."

Epp, Tracy. "Rooting for Your Health." *Vegetarian Times*, Feb, 1999, astragalus.

Granato, Heather. "Immune Function." Posted on: 09/12/2005 Virgo Publishing.

Arimoto, T., et al. "Effect of the natural antioxidant 2"-O-glycosylisovitexin on superoxide and hydroxyl radical generation." *Food Chem Toxicol.* 38(9):849-852, 2000. First Department of Medicine, Kyoto Prefectural University of Medicine, Kawaramachi Hirokoji, Kamigyo-ku, Kyoto, Japan.

Miyazaki, Y.; Tokunaga, Y.; Takagaki, K.; Tsusaki, S.; Tachibana, H.; Yamada, K. "Effect of dietary cabbage fermentation extract and young barley leaf powder on immune function of Sprague-Dawley rats." *J Nutr Sci Vitaminol* (Tokyo). 2001 Jun;47(3):253-7.
Department of Bioscience and Biotechnology, Faculty of Agriculture, Kyushu University, Fukuoka, Japan.

"Not just for Cows." Submitted by rbethini on Sun, 2006-07-16 10:28. bioscience & medicine Wheat Grass and Barley grass are full of good stuff.

Badamchian, M.; Naylor, P.H.; Spangelo, B.; Strickler, M.P.; Stone, M.J.; Hagiwara, Y.; Hagiwara, H.; and Goldstein, A.L. 1991. "Immune-endocrine Activities of Green Barley Leaf Extract (BLE): Regulation of Prolactin and Interleukin-2 Release in Vitro." *FASEB Journal*, Vol. 5, No. 4.

Kitta, K.; Hagiwara, Y.; and Shibamoto, T. 1992. "Antioxidative Activity of an Isoflavonoid, 2"-O-Glycosylisovitexin Isolated From Green Barley Leaves." *Journal of Agricultural and Food Chemistry,* Vol. 40, No. 10.

Verhoeven, D., et al. "A review of mechanisms underlying anticarcinogenicity by brassica vegetables." *Chemico-Biological Interactions*. 103(2):79-129, 1997.

Kall, M.A., et al. "Effects of dietary broccoli on human in vivo drug metabolizing enzymes: evaluation of caffeine, estrone and chlorzoxazone metabolism." *Carcinogenesis*. 17(4):793-799, 1996.

Zhang, Y., et al. "A major inducer of anticarcinogenic protective enzymes from broccoli: isolation and elucidations of structure." Proceedings of the National Academy of Sciences, USA. 89(6):2399-2403, 1992.

Thimmulappa, R.K., et al. "Identification of Nrf2-regulated genes induced by the chemopreventive agent sulforaphane by oligonucleotide microarray." *Cancer Research*. 62(18):5196-5203, 2002. Department of Environmental Health Sciences, Bloomberg School of Public Health, Johns Hopkins University, Baltimore, MA, USA.

Misiewicz, I., et al. "Sulforaphane and 2-oxohexyl isothiocyanate induce cell growth arrest and apoptosis in L-1210 leukemia and ME-18 melanoma cells." *Oncol Rep*. 10(6):2045-2050, 2003. Confocal Microscopy Laboratory, National Institute of Public Health, Warsaw, Chelmska, Poland.

Slattery, M., et al. "Carotenoids and colon cancer." *American Journal of Clinical Nutrition*. 71(2):575-582, 2000.

Fioretti, F., et al. "Risk factors for oral and pharyngeal cancer in never smokers." *Oral Oncol*. 35(4):375-378, 1999.

Enger, S.M., et al. "Dietary intake of specific carotenoids and vitamins A, C, and E, and prevalence of colorectal adenomas." *Cancer Epidemiol Biomarkers Prev*. 5(3):147-153, 1996. Department of Preventive Medicine, University of Southern California School of Medicine, Los Angeles, USA.

Raju, J.; Swamy, M.V.; Cooma, I.; Patlolla, J.M.; Pittman, B.; Reddy, B.S.; Steele, V.E.; Rao, C.V. "Low doses of beta-carotene and lutein inhibit AOM-induced rat colonic ACF formation but high doses augment ACF incidence." *Int J Cancer*. 2005 Feb 20;113(5):798-802. Chemoprevention Program, Institute For Cancer Prevention, American Health Foundation Cancer Center, Valhalla, NY, USA.

Nkondjock, A.; Ghadirian, P. "Dietary carotenoids and risk of colon cancer: case-control study." *Int J Cancer*. 2004 May 20;110(1):110-6. Epidemiology Research Unit, Research Centre, CHUM-Hotel-Dieu, Pavillon Masson, 3850 St. Urbain, Montreal, Quebec, Canada H2W 1T7.

Slattery, M.L.; Benson, J.; Curtin, K.; Ma, K.N.; Schaeffer, D.; Potter, J.D. "Carotenoids and colon cancer." *Am J Clin Nutr.* 2000 Feb;71(2):575-82. University of Utah Medical School, Salt Lake City, USA.

Tanaka, K., et al. "Augmentation of antitumor resistance by a strain of unicellular green algae, Chlorella vulgaris." *Cancer Immunol Immunother.* 17(2):90-94, 1984.

Tanaka, K., et al. "A novel glycoprotein obtained from Chlorella vulgaris strain CK22 shows antimetastatic immunopotentiation." *Cancer Immunol Immunother.* 45(6):313-320, 1998.

Hamano, K.; Gohra, H.; Katoh, T.; Fujimura, Y.; Zempo, N.; Esato, K. "The preoperative administration of lentinan ameliorated the impairment of natural killer activity after cardiopulmonary bypass." *Int J Immunopharmacol.* 1999 Aug;21(8):531-40. First Department of Surgery, Yamaguchi University School of Medicine, Ube, Japan.

Drandarska, I.; Kussovski, V.; Nikolaeva, S.; Markova, N. "Combined immunomodulating effects of BCG and Lentinan after intranasal application in guinea pigs." *Int Immunopharmacol.* 2005 Apr;5(4):795-803. Department of Immunomorphology, National Center of Infectious and Parasitic Diseases, 26, Yanko Sakazov Blvd., 1504 Sofia, Bulgaria.

Sullivan, R.; Smith, J.E.; Rowan, N.J. "Medicinal mushrooms and cancer therapy: translating a traditional practice into Western medicine." *Perspect Biol Med.* 2006 Spring;49(2):159-70. Cancer Research UK, 61 Lincoln's Inn Field, London W2A 3PX, United Kingdom.

Xiao, L.; Zhao, L.; Li, T.; Hartle, D.K.; Aruoma, O.I.; Taylor, E.W. "Activity of the dietary antioxidant ergothioneine in a virus gene-based assay for inhibitors of HIV transcription." *Biofactors.* 2006;27(1-4):157-65. Pharmaceutical and Biomedical Sciences, College of Pharmacy, University of Georgia, Athens, GA 30602 USA.

Dubost, N.; Beelman, R.; Peterson, D.; Royse, D. "Identification and quantification of ergothioneine in cultivated mushrooms by Liquid Chromatography Mass Spectroscopy." The 230th ACS National Meeting, Washington, D.C., Wednesday, August 31, 2005.

Kaila, M., et al. "Enhancement of the circulating antibody secreting response in human diarrhea by a human Lactobacillus strain." *Pediatr Res.* 32(2):141-144, 1992.

Dunne, Colum (Ph.D); Shanahan, Fergus (MD). "Role of probiotics in the treatment of intestinal infections and inflammation." *Gastrointestinal infections Current Opinion in Gastroenterology.* 18(1):40-45, January 2002.

Roberfroid, M.B. "Fructo-oligosaccharide malabsorption: benefit for gastrointestinal functions." *Curr Opin Gastroenterol.* 2000 Mar;16(2):173-7. Unite Pharmacocinetique, Metabolisme, Nutrition et Toxicologie, Brussels, Belgium.

Macfarlane, S.; Macfarlane, G.T.; Cummings, J.H. "Review article: prebiotics in the gastrointestinal tract." *Aliment Pharmacol Ther.* 2006 Sep 1;24(5):701-14. Dundee University Gut Group, Division of Pathology and Neuroscience, Ninewells Hospital and Medical School, Dundee, UK.

Clin Calcium. 2006 Oct;16(10):81-8. "Prevention of osteoporosis by foods and dietary supplements. The effect of fructooligosaccharides (FOS) on the calcium absorption and bone." Ohta A. Josai International University, Faculty of Pharmaceutical Sciences, Laboratory of Applied Nutrition.

Bengmark, S.; Gil, A. "Bioecological and nutritional control of disease: prebiotics, probiotics and synbiotics." *Nutr Hosp.* 2006 May;21 Suppl 2:72-84, 73-86. Department of Hepatology, Institute of Hepatology, University College London Medical School, 69-75 Chenies Mews, London, WC1E 6HX, United Kingdom.

Hope Smith, S., et al. "Antimutagenic activity of berry extracts." *J Med Food.* 7(4):450-455, 2004. Department of Microbiology, Clemson University, Clemson, South Carolina, USA.

Kresty, L. A., et al. "Chemoprevention of esophageal tumorigenesis by dietary administration of lyophilized black raspberries." *Cancer Research.* 61(16):6112-6119, 2001. Division of Environmental Health Sciences, School of Public Health, Comprehensive Cancer Center, The Ohio State University, Columbus, Ohio, USA.

Longnecker, M.P.; Newcomb, P.A.; Mittendorf, R., et al. "Intake of carrots, spinach, and supplements containing vitamin A in relation to risk of breast cancer." *Cancer Epidemiol Biomarkers Prev* 1997 Nov;6(11):887-92, PMID: 12980.

Penn State's College of Agricultural Sciences and the Department of Food Science provided funding for this project. Storage Time and Temperature Effects Nutrients in Spinach March 18, 2005.

Cho, M.J.; Howard, L. R. "Flavonoid content and antioxidant capacities of selected spinach genotypes determined by high-performance liquid chromatography/mass spectrometry." Dept. of Food Science, Univ. of Arkansas, 2650 N. Young Ave., Fayetteville, AR 72704

Ellinger, S.; Ellinger, J.; Stehle, P. "Tomatoes, tomato products and lycopene in the prevention and treatment of prostate cancer: do we have the evidence from intervention studies?" *Curr Opin Clin Nutr Metab Care.* 2006 Nov;9(6):722-7. aDepartment of Food and Nutrition Sciences - Nutrition Physiology bDepartment of Urology, University of Bonn, Bonn, Germany.

Giovannucci, Dr. Edward, Ph.D. Assistant Professor of Epidemiology, Department of Nutrition, Harvard University, Massachusetts. Symposium session: Epidemiology Of Prostate Cancer: Why Nutrition?

Aratanechemuge, K., et al. "Selective induction of apoptosis by ar-turmerone isolated from turmeric (Curcuma longa L) in two human leukemia cell lines, but not in human stomach cancer cell line." *Int J Mol Med.* 9(5):481-484, 2002. Faculty of Bioresources, Mie University, Tsu-city, Japan.

Azuine, M. et al. "Protective role of aqueous turmeric extract against mutagenicity of direct-acting carcinogens as well as Benzo[a]pyrene-induced genotoxicity and carcinogenicity." *J Canc Res Clin Oncol.* 118(6):447-452, 1992. Carcinogenesis Division, Tata Memorial Centre, Parel, Bombay, India.

Arora, R.B., et al. "Anti-inflammatory studies on Curcuma longa." *Ind J Med Res.* 59:1289, 1971.

Ammon, H.P.T., et al. "Mechanism of anti-inflammatory actions of curcumin and boswellic acids." *J Ethnophamacology.* 38(2-3):113-119, 1993.

Antony, S., et al. "Immunomodulatory activity of curcumin." *Immunological Investigations.* 28(5-6):291-303, 1999. Amala Cancer Research Centre, Amala Nagar, Kerala, India.

Tony Kong A-N et al., "Combined inhibitory effects of curcumin and phenethyl isothiocyanate on the growth of human PC-3 prostate xenografts in immunodeficient mice." *Cancer Research* 15 January 2006; 66 (2)

Sempertegui, F., et al. "Effects of short-term zinc supplementation on cellular immunity, respiratory symptoms, and growth of malnourished Equadorian children." *Eur J Clin Nutr.* 50(1): 42-46, 1996.

Fraker, P.J. "The dynamic link between the integrity of the immune system and zinc status." *Journal of Nutrition.* 130(5S Supplement):1399S-1406S, 2000.

Bounous, G., et al. "The immunoenhancing effect of dietary whey protein concentrate." *Clin Invest Med.* 11(4):271-278, 1988.

Meydani, S.N., et al. "Effect of vitamin E supplementation on immune responsiveness of the aged." *Annals of the New York Academy of Sciences*, USA. 570:283-290, 1989.

Nielsen, Forrest. "Nutrients keeps immune system in balance." Grand Forks Human Nutrition Resource Center, United States Agricultural Research Center, August, 2006.

Sears, William (MD); Sears, Martha (RN). "Feeding Your Immune System." http://www.askdrsears.com/about.asp

Murray, Frank. "Vitamin E can boost immune response in elderly people." *Better Nutrition* (1989-90).

Axelrod, A.E. "Role of the B vitamins in the immune response." *Adv Exp Med Biol.* 1981;135:93-106.

Carter, J. Stein. "B Vitamins and the Immune System," 1996. http://biology.clc.uc.edu/courses/bio105/vitamin.htm

De la Fuente, M. "Effects of antioxidants on immune system ageing." *Eur J Clin Nutr.* 2002 Aug;56 Suppl 3:S5-8. Departmento de Fisiologia Animal, Facultad de Ciencias Biologicas, Universidad Complutense de Madrid, Madrid, Spain.

Dhur, A.; Galan, P.; Hercberg, S. "Iron status, immune capacity and resistance to infections." *Comp Biochem Physiol A.* 1989;94(1):11-9. Institut Scientifique et Technique de l'Alimentation, Centre de Recherche sur les Anemies Nutritionnelles, Paris, France.

Alnajjar, A.; Chabane, Sari D.; Abuharfeil, N.; Hudaib, M.; Aburjai, T. "Effect of n-3 and n-6 polyunsaturated fatty acids on lymphocyte proliferation, interleukin production and phospholipid fatty acids composition in type 2 diabetic and healthy subjects in Jordan people." *Prostaglandins Leukot Essent Fatty Acids.* 2006 Jun;74(6):347-56. Epub 2006 May 2. Laboratory of Cellular Biology, Department of Biology, University of Tlemcen, P.O. Box 119, Tlemcen 13000, Algeria.

Chapter Seven – Superfoods for Weight Management & Metabolism

Berkey, Catherine S.; Rockett, Helaine R.H.; Field, Alison E.; Gillman, Matthew W.;Colditz, Graham A. "Sugar-Added Beverages and Adolescent Weight Change." *Obesity Research* 12:778-788 (2004) 2004 The North American Association for the Study of Obesity.

Fiber, by Franklin L. Murphy, MD, Franklin L. Murphy, MD, FACC, FACP, Clinical Cardiology and Internal Medicine, Clinical Professor of Medicine, UCLA School of Medicine, http://www.md-phc.com/education/fiber.html

Wien, M. *International Journal of Obesity*, November 2003; vol 27: pp. 1356-1372. Felicia Busch, RD, nutritionist, St. Paul, Minn. Michelle Wien, DrPH, RD, CDE, clinical dietitian and research fellow, City of Hope National Medical Center, Duarte, Calif. WebMD Medical News: "FDA OK's Nutty Heart Health Claim." WebMD Medical News: "Low-Carb, More Calories, Lose Weight?"

Schechter (N.D.), Steven. *Fighting Radiation & Chemical Pollutants with Foods, Herbs and Vitamins* (Vitality Books, 1997). Bee pollen, p. 80-81.

Composition of Bee Pollen, Enviro Bee Products Disributors, 5709 - 173 St. Cloverdale, B.C. V3S 4A3.

Slavin, Joanne. "Whole Grains and Human Health." *Nutrition research reviews* (2004) 17,000-000. Department of Food Science and Nutrition, University of Minnesota.

Vinson, J.A. *The Functional Food Properties of Figs.* University of Scranton, PA, February 1999, vol. 44, No. 2.

Published on Taipei Times "Sushi lovers live longer, by Michele Kirsch THE GUARDIAN, LONDON Tuesday, Apr 18, 2006, Page 16.
http://www.taipeitimes.com/News/feat/archives/2006/04/18/2003303397

Ludvik, B., et al. "Efficacy of Ipomoea batatas (Caiapo) on diabetes control in type 2 diabetic subjects treated with diet." *Diabetes Care.* 27(2):436-440, 2004.
Department of Medicine, Division of Endocrinology and Metabolism, University of Vienna, Vienna, Austria.

Beckley, Elizabeth Thompson. "American Diabetes Association Research Elicidates Link Between Weight, Fat, Carbs, and Protein." DOC News February 1, 2005, Volume 2 Number 2 p. 16 © 2005 Studies presented at North American Association for the Study of Obesity Annual Meeting.

Khan, A., et al. "Cinnamon improves glucose and lipids of people with type 2 diabetes." *Diabetes Care.* 26(12):3215-3218, 2003.

Anderson, R. A., et al. "Isolation and characterization of polyphenol type-A polymers from cinnamon with insulin-like biological activity." *J Agric Food Chem.* 52(1):65-70, 2004.

Medscape Neurology & Neurosurgery, Insomnia and Sleep Health Expert Column "The Impact of Sleep Deprivation on Hormones and Metabolism," Eve Van Cauter, PhD; Kristen Knutson, PhD; Rachel Leproult, PhD; Karine Spiegel, PhD.

"Sleep More, Eat Less," Nov. 9, 2004, CBS News By Jeanie Lerche Davis Reviewed by Brunilda Nazario, MD.

Challem, Jack; Berkson, Dr. Burton; Smith, Melissa Diane. Syndrome X, John Wiley & Sons, Inc, 2002.

Chapter Eight – Superfoods for Ligaments, Joints and Bones

Chan, Kai Ming; Anderson, Mary; Lau, Edith m.c. "Exercise Interventions: defusing the world's osteoporosis time bomb." 2003 Bulletin of the World Health Organization, 81 (11).

Food & Nutrition Research Briefs, October 2000., USDA Agricultural Research Service, Not Worth Beans.

Oxford Journals, Medicine, QJM: An International Journal of Medicine
Volume 35, Number 1, Pp. 25-38, Q J Med 1966; 35: 25-38
THE INCIDENCE OF OSTEOPOROSIS IN NORMAL WOMEN: ITS RELATION TO AGE AND MENOPAUSE, B. E. C. NORDIN2, J. MACGREGOR3 and D. A. SMITH University Department of Medicine, Gardiner Institute, Western Infirmary Glasgow, W.

Habib, K., et al. "Comparative serum cholesterol and glucose responses of rats fed on wheat flour and chickpea composite flour." *Asia Pac J Clin Nutr.* 3(Supplement):S66, 2004. Institute of Food Science and technology, University of Agriculture, Faisalabad, Pakistan.

Ott, Susan. "Bone Growth and Remolding," 2003.
http://depts.washington.edu/bonebio/ASBMRed/growth.html

NutritionData.com, calcium foods. NutritionData (ND) provides a complete nutrient analysis for any food or recipe, and helps you select foods that best match your dietary needs.

Yamori, Y.; Moriguchi, E.H.; Teramoto, T.; Miura, A.; Fukui, Y.; Honda, K.I.; Fukui, M.; Nara, Y.; Taira, K.; Moriguchi, Y. "Soybean isoflavones reduce postmenopausal bone resorption in female Japanese immigrants in Brazil: a ten-week study." *J Am Coll Nutr.* 2002 Dec;21(6):560-3. WHO Collaborating Center for Research on Primary Prevention of Cardiovascular Diseases, Kyoto, Japan. Yukio.Yamori@ma3.seikyou.ne.jp

Takada, Y.; Kobayashi, N.; Kato, K.; Matsuyama, H.; Yahiro, M.; Aoe, S. "Effects of whey protein on calcium and bone metabolism in ovariectomized rats." *J Nutr Sci Vitaminol* (Tokyo).1997 Apr;43(2):199-210. Snow Brand Milk Products Co., Ltd., Nutritional Science Laboratory, Saitama, Japan.

Fukasawa, H.; Kagechika, H.; Shudo, K. "Retinoid therapy for autoimmune diseases." *Nihon Rinsho Meneki Gakkai Kaishi.* 2006 Jun;29(3):114-26. Department of Drug Development, Institute of Medicinal and Molecular Design, Inc.

http://lpi.oregonstate.edu/infocenter/minerals/calcium/ Written by: Jane Higdon, Ph.D. Linus Pauling Institute, Oregon State University, Reviewed by: Connie M. Weaver, Ph.D. Distinguished Professor and Head of Foods and Nutrition Purdue University Last updated 04/08/2003.

Fallon, Sally; Enig PhD, Mary G. "Dem Bones: Do High Protein Diets Cause Bone Loss?" January 2000, The Weston A. Price Foundation PMB 106-380, 4200 Wisconsin Ave., NW, Washington DC 20016.

Page, Melvin E. "Degeneration, Regeneration 1949." Available from the Price Pottenger Nutrition Foundation, San Diego, CA.

E Mazariegos-Ramos et al., "Consumption of soft drinks with phosphoric acid as a risk factor for the development of hypocalcemia in children: A case control study." *Journal of Pediatrics* 1995 126:940-942.

Kimmatkar, N., et al. "Efficacy and tolerability of Boswellia serrata extract in treatment of osteoarthritis of knee - a randomized double blind placebo controlled trial." *Phytomedicine.* 10(1):3-7, 2003. MS Orthopedics, Indira Gandhi Medical College, Nagpur, India.

Etzel, R. "Special extract of boswellia serrata (H 15) in the treatment of rheumatoid arthritis." *Phytomedicine.* 3(1):91-94, 1996.

Singh, G.B., et al. "Pharmacology of an extract of salai guggal ex-Boswellia serrata, a new non-steroidal anti-inflammatory agent." *Agents Actions.* 18(3-4):407-412, 1986.

Ammon, H.P. "Boswellic acids in chronic inflammatory diseases." *Planta Med.* 2006 Oct;72(12):1100-16. Dept. of Pharmacology, Institute of Pharmaceutical Sciences, University of Tuebingen, Tuebingen, Germany. sekretariat.ammon@uni-tuebingen.de

Chopra, A. Lavin, P.; Patwardhan, B.; Chitre, D. "A 32-Week Randomized, Placebo-Controlled Clinical Evaluation of RA-11, an Ayurvedic Drug, on Osteoarthritis of the Knees." *J Clin Rheumatol.* 2004 Oct;10(5):236-245. From the *Center for Rheumatic Diseases, Inlaks and Budhrani Hospital, Bharati Hospital Medical College (Deemed University), Pune, India; daggerAverion, Inc., Framingham, Massachusetts; the Double Dagger School of Health Sciences, University of Pune, India; and section sign BIO-VED Pharmaceuticals, Inc., San Jose, California.

Ojewole, J.A. "Analgesic, antiinflammatory and hypoglycaemic effects of ethanol extract of Zingiber officinale (Roscoe) rhizomes (Zingiberaceae) in mice and rats." *Phytother Res.* 2006 Sep;20(9):764-72. Department of Pharmacology, Faculty of Health Sciences, University of KwaZulu-Natal, Private Bag X54001, Durban, South Africa. ojewolej@ukzn.ac.za

Srivastava, K.C., et al. "Ginger (Zingiber officinale) in rheumatism and musculoskeletal disorders." *Med Hypotheses.* 39(4):342-348, 1992.

Altman, R.D., et al. "Effects of ginger extract on knee pain in patients with osteoarthritis." *Arthritis Rheum.* 44(11):2531-2538, 2001.

Grzanna, R.; Lindmark, L.; Frondoza, C.G. *J Med Food.* "Ginger--an herbal medicinal product with broad anti-inflammatory actions." 2005 Summer;8(2):125-32. RMG Biosciences,Inc.

Funk J.L.; Oyarzo, J.N.; Frye, J.B.; Chen, G.; Lantz, R.C.; Jolad, S.D.; Solyom, A.M.; Timmermann, B.N. "Turmeric extracts containing curcuminoids prevent experimental rheumatoid arthritis." *J Nat Prod.* 2006 Mar;69(3):351-5. Arizona Center for Phytomedicine Research, Department of Medicine, Department of Cell Biology and Anatomy, University of Arizona, Tucson, 85724, USA.

Meacham, S.L.; Taper, L.J.; Volpe, S.L. "Effect of boron supplementation on blood and urinary calcium, magnesium, and phosphorus, and urinary boron in athletic and sedentary women." *American Journal of Clinical Nutrition.* 61(2):341-345,1995.

Chapin, R.E., et al. "The effects of dietary boric acid on bone strength in rats." *Biol Trace Elem Res.* 66(1-3):395-399, 1998.

Chapin, R.E., et al. "The effects of dietary boron on bone strength in rats." *Fundam Appl Toxicol.* 35(2):205-215, 1997. Reproductive Toxicology Group, NIEHS, Research Triangle Park, North Carolina, USA.

Orihuela, D.; Meichtry, V.; Pizarro, M. "Aluminium-induced impairment of transcellular calcium absorption in the small intestine: calcium uptake and glutathione influence." *J Inorg Biochem.* 2005 Sep;99(9):1879-86. Laboratorio de Investigaciones Fisiologicas Experimentales, Facultad de Bioquimica y Ciencias Biologicas, Universidad Nacional del Litoral, Piso 4, Ciudad Universitaria, Paraje El Pozo (3000) Santa Fe, Argentina.

Weaver, C.M., et al. "Oxalic acid decreases calcium absorption in rats." *Journal of Nutrition.* 117(11):1903-1906, 1987.

Fredlund, K.: Isaksson, M.; Rossander-Hulthen, L.; Almgren, A.; Sandberg, A.S. "Absorption of zinc and retention of calcium: dose-dependent inhibition by phytate." *J Trace Elem Med Biol.* 2006;20(1):49-57. Epub 2006 Mar 2. Department of Chemical and Biological Engineering/Food Science, Chalmers University of Technology, SE 412 96, Goteborg, Sweden.

Bjorneboe, G.E., et al. "Calcium status and calcium-regulating hormones in alcoholics." *Alcoholism.* 12(2):229-232, 1988.

Kruger, M.C.; Horrobin, D.F. "Calcium metabolism, osteoporosis and essential fatty acids: a review." *Prog Lipid Res.* 1997 Sep;36(2-3):131-51. Department of Physiology, University of Pretoria, South Africa.

Claassen, N.; Coetzer, H.; Steinmann, C.M.; Kruger, M.C. "The effect of different n-6/n-3 essential fatty acid ratios on calcium balance and bone in rats." *Prostaglandins Leukot Essent Fatty Acids.* 1995 Jul;53(1):13-9. Department of Physiology, Faculty of Medicine, University of Pretoria, South Africa.

Simopoulos, A.P. "Evolutionary aspects of diet, the omega-6/omega-3 ratio and genetic variation: nutritional implications for chronic diseases." *Biomed Pharmacother.* 2006 Nov;60(9):502-507. Epub 2006 Aug 28. The Center for Genetics, Nutrition and Health, 2001 S Street, NW, Suite 530, 20009 Washington, DC, USA.

Maroon, J.C.; Bost, J.W. "Omega-3 fatty acids (fish oil) as an anti-inflammatory: an alternative to nonsteroidal anti-inflammatory drugs for discogenic pain." *Surg Neurol.* 2006 Apr;65(4):326-31. Comment in: Surg Neurol. 2006 Apr;65(4):325. Department of Neurological Surgery, University of Pittsburgh Medical Center, Pittsburgh, PA, USA.

Ghosh, P.; Shimmon, S.; Whitehouse, M.W. "Arthritic disease suppression and cartilage protection with glycosaminoglycan polypeptide complexes (Peptacans) derived from the cartilage extracellular matrix: a novel approach to therapy." *Inflammopharmacology.* 2006 Aug;14(3-4):155-62. Institute for Nutraceutical Research, PO Box 35, Brookvale, New South Wales, 2100, Australia.

Chan, P.S.; Caron, J.P.; Orth, M.W. "Short-term gene expression changes in cartilage explants stimulated with interleukin beta plus glucosamine and chondroitin sulfate." *J Rheumatol.* 2006 Jul;33(7):1329-40. Bone and Joint Center, Henry Ford Hospital, Michigan, USA.

Parelman, M.; Stoecker, B.; Baker, A.; Medeiros, D. "Iron restriction negatively affects bone in female rats and mineralization of hFOB osteoblast cells." *Exp Biol Med* (Maywood). 2006 Apr;231(4):378-86. Department of Human Nutrition, Kansas State University, Manhattan, KS 66506, USA.

Harris, Margaret M.; Houtkooper, Linda B.; Stanford, Vanessa A.; Parkhill, Carly; Weber, Judith L.; Flint-Wagner, Hilary; Weiss, Lauren; Going, Scott B.; Lohman, Timothy G. "Nutrition and Aging, Dietary Iron Is Associated with Bone Mineral Density in Healthy Postmenopausal Women." *The American Society for Nutritional Sciences J. Nutr.* 133:3598-3602, November 2003 Department of Physiology and Department of Nutritional Sciences, The University of Arizona, Tucson, AZ 85721; Department of Pediatrics, Center for Applied Research and Evaluation, University of Arkansas for Medical Sciences, Little Rock, AR 72202; Department of Health and Behavior Studies, Teachers College, Columbia University, New York, NY.

Nielsen, F.H. "A mild magnesium deprivation affects calcium excretion but not bone strength and shape, including changes induced by nickel deprivation, in the rat." *Biol Trace Elem Res.* 2006 May;110(2):133-50. US Department of Agriculture, Agricultural Research Service, Grand Forks Human Nutrition Research Center, Grand Forks, ND 58202-9034, USA.

Shapiro, R., et al. "Co-dependence of calcium and phosphorus for growth and bone development under conditions of varying deficiency." *Bone.* 32(5):532-540, 2003.

Borek, C. "Bone up on osteoporosis." *Nutrition Science News.* November 2000. Potassium facilitates the retention of calcium by the kidneys and thereby helps to prevent calcium loss.

Macdonald, H.M., et al. "Low dietary potassium intakes and high dietary estimates of net endogenous acid production are associated with low bone mineral density in premenopausal women and increased markers of bone resorption in postmenopausal women." *Am J Clin Nutr.* 81(4):923-933, 2005. Department of Medicine and Therapeutics, University of Aberdeen, Medical School Buildings, Aberdeen, United Kingdom.

Hannan, M.T.; Tucker, K.L.; Dawson-Hughes, B.; Cupples, L.A.; Felson, D.T.; Kiel, D.P. "Effect of dietary protein on bone loss in elderly men and women: the Framingham Osteoporosis Study." *J Bone Miner Res.* 2000 Dec;15(12):2504-12. Hebrew Rehabilitation Center for Aged, Research and Training Institute and Harvard Medical School Division on Aging, Boston, Massachusetts 02131-1097, USA.

Sasaki, S.; Iwata, H.; Ishiguro, N.; Habuchi, O.; Miura, T. Low-selenium diet, bone, and articular cartilage in rats. *Nutrition.* 1994 Nov-Dec;10(6):538-43. Department of Orthopedic Surgery, Nagoya University School of Medicine, Japan.

Yazar, M.; Sarban, S.; Kocyigit, A.; Isikan, U.E. Synovial fluid and plasma selenium, copper, zinc, and iron concentrations in patients with rheumatoid arthritis and Osteoarthritis. *Biol Trace Elem Res.* 2005 Aug;106(2):123-32. Department of Orthopaedic Surgery, Harran University, Medical Faculty, 63200 Sanliurfa-Turkey.

Kurz, B., et al. "Dietary vitamins and selenium diminish the development of mechanically induced osteoarthritis and increase the expression of antioxidative enzymes in the knee joint of STR/1N mice." *Osteoarthritis Cartilage.* 10(2):119-126, 2002.

Jugdaohsingh, R.; Tucker, K.L.; Qiao, N.; Cupples, L.A.; Kiel, D.P.; Powell, J.J. "Dietary silicon intake is positively associated with bone mineral density in men and premenopausal women of the Framingham Offspring cohort." *J Bone Miner Res.* 2004 Feb;19(2):297-307. Epub 2003 Dec 16. Gastrointestinal Laboratory, The Rayne Institute, St Thomas' Hospital, London, United Kingdom.

Malladi, P.; Xu, Y.; Yang, G.P.; Longaker, M.T. "Functions of vitamin D, retinoic acid, and dexamethasone in mouse adipose-derived mesenchymal cells." *Tissue Eng.* 2006 Jul;12(7):2031-40. Children's Surgical Research Program, Department of Surgery, Stanford University School of Medicine, Stanford, California 94305, USA.

Cockayne, S.; Adamson, J.; Lanham-New, S.; Shearer, M.J.; Gilbody, S.; Torgerson, D.J. "Vitamin K and the prevention of fractures: systematic review and meta-analysis of randomized controlled trials." *Arch Intern Med.* 2006 Jun 26;166(12):1256-61. York Trials Unit, Department of Health Sciences, University of York, York YO10 5DD, England.

Yamaguchi, M., et al. "Receptor activator of NF-kappaB ligand-stimulated osteoclastogenesis in mouse marrow culture is suppressed by zinc in vitro." *Int J Mol Med.* 14(1):81-85, 2004. Laboratory of Endocrinology and Molecular Metabolism, Graduate School of Nutritional Sciences, University of Shizuoka, Shizuoka, Japan.

Peretz. A., et al. "Zinc supplementation increases bone alkaline phosphatase in healthy men." *J Trace Elem Med Biol.* 15(2-3):175-178, 2001. Department of Rheumatology, Brugmann University Hospital, Brussels, Belgium.

Lowe, N.M., et al. "Is there a potential therapeutic value of copper and zinc for osteoporosis?" *Proc Nutr Soc.* 61(2):181-185, 2002. Department of Biological Sciences, University of Central Lancashire, Preston, UK.

Cerhan, J.R., et al. "Antioxidant micronutrients and risk of rheumatoid arthritis in a cohort of older women." *American Journal of Epidemiology.* 157(4):345-354, 2003. Department of Health Sciences Research, Mayo Clinic, Rochester, MN.

Balogh, Z., et al. "Plasma zinc and its relationship to clinical symptoms and drug treatment in rheumatoid arthritis." *Ann Rheum Dis.* 39(4):329032, 1980.

"B Vitamins May Cut Fracture Risk After Stroke," by Serena Gordon, HealthDay Reporter Source: Yoshihiro Sato, M.D., President, Department of Neurology, Mitate Hospital, Tagawa, and Professor, Hirosaki University School of Medicine, Hirosaki, Japan; Joyce van Meurs, Ph.D., Senior Researcher, Department of Internal Medicine and Epidemiology and Diostatistics, Erasmus Medical Center, Rotterdam, the Netherlands; March 2, 2005, *Journal of the American Medical Association.*

"Yoga Is More Effective Than Conventional Exercise For Back Pain, Group Health Study Finds," January 3, 2006, Group Health Cooperative Center for Health Studies, Science Daily News.

Ernst E. "Complementary or alternative therapies for osteoarthritis." *Nat Clin Pract Rheumatol.* 2006 Feb;2(2):74-80. Complementary Medicine Peninsula Medical School, Universities of Exeter & Plymouth, UK.

Chapter Nine-Superfoods for Skin, Hair and Nails

The Avocado and Human Nutrition. I. Some Human Health Aspects of the Avocado Bob Bergh, Department of Botany and Plant Sciences, University of California, Riverside, CA 92521, USA.

Solovchenko, Alexei and Schmitz-Eiberger, Michaela. "Significance of skin flavonoids for UV-B-protection in apple fruits." *Journal of Experimental Botany*, Vol. 54, No. 389, pp. 1977-1984, August 1, 2003 © 2003 Oxford University Press. 1 Department of Physiology of Microorganisms, Faculty of Biology, Moscow State University, GSP-2 Moscow 119992, Russia, Department of Horticulture, Bonn University, Auf dem Hügel 6, D-53121 Bonn, Germany.

NutritionData.com, brazil nuts, cashews, pistachio nuts, walnuts and sunflower seeds. NutritionData (ND) provides a complete nutrient analysis for any food or recipe, and helps you select foods that best match your dietary needs.

September 2006 issue of *Healthy Food Guide*, by Sharon Natoli is an accredited practising dietitian with Food and Nutrition Australia.

Dinkova-Kostova, A.T.; Jenkins, S.N.; Fahey, J.W.; Ye, L.; Wehage, S.L.; Liby, K.T.; Stephenson, K.K.; Wade, K.L.; Talalay, P. "Protection against UV-light-induced skin carcinogenesis in SKH-1 high-risk mice by sulforaphane-containing broccoli sprout extracts." *Cancer Lett.* 2006 Aug 28;240(2):243-52. Epub 2005 Nov 3. The Lewis B. and Dorothy Cullman Cancer Chemoprotection Center, Department of Pharmacology and Molecular Sciences, School of Medicine, Johns Hopkins University, 725 N. Wolfe Street, Baltimore, MD 21205, USA.

NutritionData.com, brussel sprouts, green peas, kiwi, shrimp. NutritionData (ND) provides a complete nutrient analysis for any food or recipe, and helps you select foods that best match your dietary needs.

O'Byrne, Dawn J.; Devaraj, Scidevi; Grundy, Scott M.; Jialal, Ishwarlal. "Comparison of the antioxidant effects of Concord grape juice flavonoids and a-tocopherol on markers of oxidative stress in healthy adults." *Am J Clin Nutr.* 2002;1367-74.

Scheer, James F. "Silica: health and beauty from nature." *Better Nutrition*, Dec, 1997.

Carlisle, E.M. "Silicon as an Essential Trace Element in Animal Nutrition." In: Silicon Biochemistry. CIBA Foundation Symposium 121. New York: John Wiley & Sons, 1986.

Calomme, M.R., et al. "Supplementation of calves with stabilized orthosilicic acid. Effect on the Silicon, Ca, Mg, and P concentrations in serum and the collagen concentration in skin and cartilage." *Biol Trace Elem Res.* 56(2):153-165. 1997.

Better Nutrition, March, 1999 Red clover Kathi Keville.

University of Maryland Medical Center, Center for Integrative Medicine, Red Clover, http://www.umm.edu/altmed/ConsHerbs/RedCloverch.html

Ayres, S. Jr., et al. "Acne vulgaris and lipid peroxidation: new concepts in pathogenesis and treatment." *International Journal of Dermatology.* 17:305, 1978.

Kligman, A.M., et al. "Oral vitamin A in acne vulgaris." *Int J Dermatol.* 20:278-285, 1981.

Ji, H.G., et al. "Retinyl palmitate at 5 percent in a cream: its stability, efficacy and effect." *Cosmet Toil.* 114:61-68, 1999.

Strosser, A.V., et al. "Synthetic vitamin A in the treatment of eczema in children." *Annals Allergy.* 10:703-704, 1952.

Varani, J., et al. "Vitamin A antagonizes decreased cell growth and elevated collagen-degrading matrix metalloproteinases and stimulates collagen accumulation in naturally aged human skin." *J Invest Dermatol.* 114(3):480-486, 2000. Departments of Pathology and Dermatology, The University of Michigan, Medical School, Ann Arbor, MI, USA.

Pearson, D. & Shaw, S. *The Life Extension Companion.* Warner Books, New York, USA, 1984:88-89.

Haas, Elson M. Staying Healthy with Nutrition. Celestial Arts, Berkeley, California, USA. 1992:116. Vitamin B2 is often used to treat acne.

Blanck. H.M., et al. "Angular stomatitis and riboflavin status among adolescent Bhutanese refugees living in southeastern Nepal." *American Journal of Clinical Nutrition.* 76(2):430-435, 2002.

Lo, C.S., et al. "Riboflavin status of adolescents in southern China. Average intake of riboflavin and clinical findings." *Med J Aust.* 141(10):635-637, 1984.

Namazi, M.R., et al. "Nicotinamide: a potential addition to the anti-psoriatic weaponry." *FASEB J.* 17(11):1377-1379, 2003. Dermatology Department, Shiraz University of Medical Sciences, Shiraz, Iran.

Leung, L.H. "Pantothenic acid deficiency as the pathogenesis of acne vulgaris." *Medical Hypotheses.* 44:490-492, 1995.

Kelly, G.S., et al. "Pantethine: a review of its biochemistry and therapeutic applications." *Alternative Medicine Review.* 2(5):365-377, 1997. Vitamin B5 deficiency in animals can cause dermatitis.

Holman, P. "Pyridoxine   vitamin B-6." *Journal of the Australasian College of Nutritional and Environmental Medicine.* 14(1), 1995.

Snider, B., et al. "Pyridoxine therapy for premenstrual acne flare." *Arch Dermatol.* 110:130-131, 1974.

Charles, B.M., et al. "Biotin-responsive alopecia and developmental regression." *Lancet.* 2(8134):118-120, 1979.

Floersheim, G.L. "Treatment of brittle fingernails with biotin." *Z Hautkr.* 64(1):41-48, 1989.

Colombo, V.E., et al. "Treatment of brittle fingernails and onychoschizia with biotin: scanning electron microscopy." *J Am Acad Dermatol.* 23(6 Part 1):1127-1132, 1990.

Lassus, A. "Colloidal silicic acid for oral and topical treatment of aged skin, fragile hair and brittle nails in females." *J Int Med Res.* 21(4):209-215, 1993.

Calomme, M.R., et al. "Supplementation of calves with stabilized orthosilicic acid. Effect on the silicon, Ca, Mg, and P concentrations in serum and the collagen concentration in skin and cartilage." *Biol Trace Elem Res.* 56(2):153-165. 1997.

Ranjbar, A., et al. "Selenium and atopic dermatitis - systemic treatment with sodium selenite, a new therapeutical concept for the treatment of atopic dermatitis in children." *International Pediatrics.* 16(2):96, 2001.

Juhlin, L., et al. "Blood glutathione-peroxidase levels in skin diseases: Effect of selenium and vitamin E treatment." *Acta Dermatovener* (Stockholm). 62(3):211-214, 1982.

Dreno, B., et al. "Zinc salts effects on granulocyte zinc concentration and chemotaxis in acne patients." *Acta Derm Venereol.* 72(4):250-252, 1992.

Cunliff, W.J., et al. "A double-blind trial of a zinc sulphate/zinc citrate complex and tetracycline in the treatment of acne." *British Journal of Dermatology.* 101(3):321-325, 1979.

Rostan, E.F., et al. :Evidence supporting zinc as an important antioxidant for skin." *International Journal of Dermatology.* 41(9):606-611, 2002. Duke University, Durham, NC, and SkinCeuticals, Dallas, TX, USA.

Segala, M. (editor). *Disease Prevention and Treatment* 3rd Edition. Life Extension Media. Florida, USA. 2000:690.

Eck, Dr. Paul C.; Wilson, Dr. Larry. "Hair Loss, A Growing Concern." The Eck Institute of Applied Nutrition and Bioenergetics, Ltd.

Bjerve, K.S., et al. "Alpha-linolenic acid deficiency in patients on long-term gastric-tube feeding: Estimation of linolenic acid and long-chain unsaturated n-3 fatty acid requirement in man." *American Journal of Clinical Nutrition.* 45:66, 1987.

Galland, L. "Increased requirements for essential fatty acids in atopic individuals: a review with clinical descriptions." *J Am Coll Nutr.* 5(2):213-228, 1986.

Vahlquist, C., et al. "The fatty-acid spectrum in plasma and adipose tissue in patients with psoriasis." *Archives of Dermatology Research.* 278(2):114-119, 1985.

Smart Skin Biology, http://www.smartskincare.com/skinbiology

Fitzgerald, Dr. Patricia. *The Detox Solution*, Illumination Press, 2001, pp. 91 309, 318.

Human Physiology/Integumentary System,
 http://en.wikibooks.org/wiki/Human_Physiology/Integumentary_System#Hair

References and Informational Websites

About Polyphenolics
http://www.polyphenolics.com
- *Good information on grape seed extracts from a wine producer. Polyphenolics conducts in-house research, and maintains close affiliations and working partnerships with respected universities and research institutions worldwide.*

American Journal of Clinical Nutrition
http://www.ajcn.org/current.shtml
- *Excellent references for past and current research projects in the nutritional field.*

American Obesity Association
http://www.obesity.org/education
- *Latest news and studies on obesity in America.*

Ask Dr. Bill Sears
http://www.askdrsears.com
- *Dr. Sears, a pediatric doctor and his wife Martha, an RN. Have been practicing pediatric medicine for more than 30 years. Their website is filled with information on nutrition for children. This is one of my favorite websites!*

Bastyr Center for Natural Health
http://www.bastyrcenter.org
- *Bastyr Center for Natural Health is the largest natural health clinic in the state of Washington and is the teaching clinic of Bastyr University, which is a leading expert in natural medicine.*

Beyond Vegetarianism
http://www.beyondveg.com
- *Great information about vegetarian, vegan and raw-food diets from long-time insiders.*

Brain Power
http://www.smart-kit.com
- *A website dedicated to brain enhancement.*

Clinical Trials.gov
http://clinicaltrials.gov
- *ClinicalTrials.gov provides regularly updated information about federally and privately supported clinical research in human volunteers.*

Dr. David Williams, Heart Health
http://www.drdavidwilliams.com
- *A great website with information on alterative health. Dr. Williams has traveled worldwide to locate, evaluate, formulate, and write about proven treatments and cures for practically every major health concern today.*

Entrez PubMed
http://www.ncbi.nlm.nih.gov
- *PubMed is a service of the U.S. National Library of Medicine that includes over 16 million citations from MEDLINE and other life science journals for biomedical articles back to the 1950s. PubMed includes links to full text articles and other related resources.*

FCIC Health
http://www.pueblo.gsa.gov
- *Federal Citizens Information Center.*

Functional Foods and Nutraceuticals
http://www.ffnmag.com
- *Information on the latest trends in nutraceuticals.*

Functional Foods Glossary
http://www.arfunctionalfoods.org
- *The Functional Foods of the Mid-South project goal was to systematically investigate the development and health benefits of functional foods derived from economically important, phytonutrient-rich Mid-South crops, such as spinach, blueberries, rice and soybeans.*

Harvard Gazette Science
http://www.news.harvard.edu
- *Harvard's Office of News and Public Affairs is the liaison between the University and the news media and the general public.*

Health Benefits of Yoga
http://www.abc-of-yoga.com
- *Welcome to your complete resource of Yoga information. ABC of Yoga covers a wide range of topics about the different aspects of the practice such as the various styles, postures, poses, and techniques.*

Health Science Institute
http://www.hsibaltimore.com/
- *Information on alternative health.*

Health World Online
http://www.healthy.net
- *Resource on wellness, natural health, traditional, complementary and alternative medicine information, and self care.*

Herb Med
http://www.herbmed.org
- *Provides hyperlinked access to the scientific data underlying the use of herbs for health.*

Herbal Safety
http://www.herbalsafety.utep.edu
> • *Facts and safety information presented by the University of Texas, El Paso.*

Kids Health for Parents
http://www.kidshealth.org
> • *Up-to-date information on growth, food and fitness, childhood infections, immunizations, and medical conditions from the Nemours foundation.*

Linus Pauling Institute
http://lpi.oregonstate.edu/infocenter
> • *Source for current scientific information regarding roles of specific vitamins, minerals, and other nutrients in preventing disease and promoting health.*

Living Beyond Breast Cancer
http://www.lbbc.org
> • *Dedicated to empowering all affected by this disease. Includes a newsletter, transcripts and an email list. Headquartered in Ardmore, Pennsylvania.*

Medical Library
http://www.medical-library.net
> • *Introduction to the Doctors' Medical Library.*

Medicine Net.com
http://www.medicinenet.com
> • *Patient-focused site covering over 400 conditions and diseases, more than 100 tests and procedures, and a medical dictionary of more than 6,500 terms.*

Merck Manuals Online Medical Library
http://www.merck.com/mrkshared/mmanual/home.jsp
> • *Excellent resource on health issues.*

National Center for Complementary and Alternative Medicine
http://nccam.nih.gov/
> • *Resource on complementary and alternative medicine.*

New England Journal of Medicine
http://content.nejm.org
> • *Peer-reviewed medical journal online featuring current medical research information, reviews and articles for biomedical science and internal medicine.*

Nutra Ingredients
http://www.nutraingredients-usa.com
> • *Daily news on nutritional supplements, energy drinks, sport nutrition and vitamins. Free access to news on health food in North America.*

Nutrient Data
http://www.ars.usda.gov
- *The main in-house research arm of the US Department of Agriculture. Research news, find-a-researcher, consumer and educational information on a wide range.*

Nutrition Data.
http://www.nutritiondata.com
- *Nutrition facts, calorie counter and calculator promotes healthy eating by telling you, in simple terms, what is good and bad about the foods you eat.*

P&G Hair Care Research Center
http://www.pg.com/science/haircare
- *The World of Hair, an on-line reference by Dr. John Gray, provided by the P&G Hair Care Research Center.*

Pam Rotella, Vegetarian Fun
http://www.pamrotella.com
- *A long-time vegetarian and author of Vegan Vegetarian Cooking, Rotella has great information.*

Phytochemicals
http://www.phytochemicals.info
- *Explains in detail all about phytochemicals.*

Shirley's Wellness Cafe
http://www.shirleys-wellness-cafe.com
- *Oriented to self care, a free educational web site dedicated to help promote natural health for humans and their animals.*

Sloan-Kettering Cancer Center
http://www.mskcc.org/mskcc/html/11570.cfm
- *Great information on herbal medicine.*

Smart Skin Care
http://www.smartskincare.com
- *Skin care and rejuvenation information and reviews based on published research and other independent sources.*

The World's Healthiest Foods
http://www.whfoods.com
- *Non-profit foundation providing reliable, scientifically accurate, personalized information for convenient and enjoyable healthy eating.*

University Davis Health Systems
http://www.ucdmc.ucdavis.edu
- *University of California system comprised of the Medical Center and School of Medicine. Educational programs for health professionals.*

University of Maryland Medical Center
http://www.umm.edu
  • *Resources on health and wellness.*

Vegetarian Nutrition
http://www.andrews.edu
  • *The flagship educational institution of the Seventh-day Adventist Church.*

Vitamin Herb University
http://www.vitaminherbuniversity.com
  • *Resource education on dietary supplements, vitamin information and herb information, and drug herb interaction.*

Glossary

Acetylcholine: participates in the transmission of nerve impulses at different parts of the body and is found in both the central nervous system, where it passes signals between neurons, and in the peripheral nervous system, where it relays nerve impulses from motor nerves to muscles.

Amino Acids: These compounds are the building blocks of proteins and contain either a carbon, hydrogen, oxygen, nitrogen, and in certain cases sulfur. They are characterized by the presence of a carboxyl group (COOH) and an amino group (NH_2) attached to the same carbon at the end of the compound.

Amino Acids (Essential): An amino acid that is required by animals but that they cannot synthesize; must be supplied in the diet. Eight amino acids are generally regarded as essential for humans: tryptophan, lysine, methionine, phenylalanine, threonine, valine, leucine, and isoleucine. Two others, histidine and arginine are essential only in children and possibly seniors.

Anthocyanins: These represent a group of phytonutrients within the larger category called "phenolics." Anthocyanins give intense color to certain red and/or blue fruits and vegetables. These plant pigments are very powerful antioxidants and have been studied extensively for their ability to fight heart disease and cancer and to delay several diseases associated with the aging process.

Antigens: These are any foreign substance that when introduced into the body stimulates the production of an antibody. Antigens include toxins, bacteria, foreign blood cells, and the cells of transplanted organs.

Antioxidants: Antioxidants are found naturally in many fruits and vegetables and act to protect cells from damage caused by the by-products (free-radicals) of everyday metabolism and toxic substances in the environment and food. Over time, free radicals can significantly damage cells and lead to a number of diseases associated with aging. Antioxidants act as little vacuum cleaners, eliminating free radicals as they circulate throughout the body, preventing them from doing damage to substance that inhibits oxidation or inhibits reactions promoted by oxygen or peroxides.

Appestat: The area in the brain that is believed to regulate appetite and food intake.

Beta-glucan: Beta glucans are polysaccharides (sugar molecules) found bound together as a sugar/protein complex. The richest concentrated source of beta glucan is baker's yeast cell walls, but it is also present in lesser amounts in barley, oats, and some seaweeds, mushrooms and other plants.

Beta-sitosterol: β-sitosterol is one of several phytosterols with chemical structures similar to that of cholesterol and has been found to lower blood cholesterol levels in the body by blocking absorption of cholesterol in your bloodstream. It is white in color and waxy in nature and widely distributed in the plant kingdom.

Bifidobacteria: These are one of the major strains of bacteria that make up the gut flora, the bacteria that reside in the colon and have health benefits for their hosts.

Bioflavonoids: These are a subcategory of the phytonutrients flavonoids, found in citrus fruits and are antioxidants that help prevent cancer-causing hormones from attaching to the body's cells. They are especially protecting of the eyes and nerves and help with symptoms of allergies, arthritis and asthma.

Biotin: Biotin is a water-soluble B-complex vitamin important in the catalysis of essential metabolic reactions to synthesize fatty acids, cell growth, metabolism of fats, and amino acids. It plays a role in the Krebs Cycle, which is the process in which energy is released from food. It is also indicated for healthy hair and skin, healthy sweat glands, nerve tissue, and bone marrow, and assisting with muscle pain. It helps with the transfer of carbon dioxide and in maintaining a steady blood sugar level.

Carotenoids: Carotenoids are powerful antioxidants providing protection against oxidative damage, and they stimulate immune function. Persons with high levels of serum carotenoids have a reduced risk of heart disease and cancer. Carotenoids are the pigments found in yellow-orange, red, and green vegetables and the yellow-orange fruits.

Carminative: An agent that prevents or relieves flatulence (gas in the gastrointestinal tract).

Catechin: Catechin are bioflavonoids, polyphenols and powerful anti-oxidants found in white tea, green tea and cocoa. Catechins are linked to evidence of fighting tumors as well as enhancing immune system function, due to their polyphenol antioxidant character. Catechins are capable of crossing the body's blood-brain barrier (due to the fact that they are both water-soluble and fat-soluble). This permits catechins to influence brain function.

Carbohydrates: These provide fuel for the body and are an important part of a healthy, balanced diet. They include sugars, fibers and starches found in various foods. The digestive system breaks carbohydrates down into single sugar molecules so they can be absorbed into the bloodstream. It also converts most digestible carbohydrates into glucose (also known as blood sugar), which our cells use as a universal energy source. Simple or fast-acting carbohydrates include fruit juices and refined white bread and rice. Complex carbohydrates, which take longer to break down in the body, include whole grains, fruits and vegetables.

Cholesterol: A waxy, fat-like substance made in the liver, and found in the blood and in all cells of the body. It's important for good health and is needed for making cell walls, tissues, hormones, vitamin D, and bile acid. Cholesterol also comes from eating foods taken from animals such as egg yolks, meat, and whole-milk dairy products.

Choline: This is a nutrient, essential for cardiovascular and brain function, and for cellular membrane (comprising 33%) composition and repair. The foods richest in phosphatidylcholine–the major delivery form of choline–are lecithin, beef, beef liver, egg yolks, pork and soy.

Chondroitin: This is usually found attached to proteins as part of a proteoglycan. Chondroitin sulfate is a major structural component of cartilage and provides much of its resistance to compression. Along with glucosamine, chondroitin sulfate has become a widely used dietary supplement for treatment of osteoarthritis.

Conjugated Linoleic Acid (CLA): Refers to group of modified forms of linoleic acid found in dairy products and meat. Many studies on CLA in humans show a tendency for reduced body fat, particularly abdominal fat, changes in serum total lipids and decreased whole body glucose uptake. Dietary CLA supplementation does not seem to have any adverse effects. The maximum reduction in body fat mass was achieved with a 3.4 g daily dose split into three divided doses throughout the day. Food products of grass-fed lamb or beef are good sources of CLA.

Coenzyme Q10 (CoQ10): One of the best-known effects of this compound is its antioxidant qualities as well as the control it exercises on the flow of oxygen within cells, assistance with cardiovascular functioning, the production of energy, its assistance with absorption of other nutrients as well as its immune boosting properties. It is used to produce energy to fuel cell growth and maintenance. The highest amounts of coenzyme Q10 are in the heart, liver, kidneys, and pancreas and the lowest amounts are in the lungs. The levels of coenzyme Q10 normally decline with age.

Cruciferous: This is known as the mustard family or cabbage family of plants, encompassing the cabbage, brussels sprouts, broccoli, kohlrabi, cauliflower, kale, and most recently broccoflower, a hybrid of broccoli and cauliflower. This family of plants is known for its anti-cancer properties.

Cytokines: These are a group of signaling compounds that, like hormones and neurotransmitters, are used extensively for inter-cell communication. They are critical to the functioning of both innate and adaptive immune responses. Apart from their importance in the development and functioning of the immune system, cytokines play a major role in a variety of immunological, inflammatory and infectious diseases.

Docosahexaenoic Acid (DHA): An essential fatty acid, is most often found in fish oil. Most animals make very little DHA metabolically, however small amounts are manufactured internally through the consumption of α-linolenic acid, an omega-3 fatty acid found in chia, flax, and many other seeds and nuts. DHA is a major fatty acid in sperm and brain phospholipids, especially in the retina. Dietary DHA can reduce the level of blood triglycerides. Low levels of DHA cause reduction of brain serotonin levels and have been associated with ADHD, Alzheimer's disease, and depression, among other diseases, and there is mounting evidence that DHA supplementation may be effective in combating such diseases.

Dimethylethanolamine (DMAE): DMAE is related to choline and is a biochemical precursor to the neurotransmitter acetylcholine, and found naturally in fishes like sardines and anchovies. Consumption of DMAE have shown an increase in alertness, with a positive influence on mood.

Dietary Reference Intakes (DRI): A joint collaboration with Canada and the US, DRIs are revised recommendations for vitamins and minerals from the Institute of Medicine, an arm of the National Academy of Sciences, which will gradually replace the Recommended Dietary Allowances or RDA guidelines. DRIs are being developed for vitamins and minerals that currently have no RDAs.

Duodenum: In anatomy of the digestive system, the duodenum is a hollow jointed tube connecting the stomach to the jejunum. It is the first and shortest part of the small intestine and is mainly responsible for the breakdown of food in the small intestine.

Daily Value (DV): A term on food labels based on the RDA, designed to help consumers use food label information to plan a healthy diet. Usually based on a 2,000 calorie a day diet.

Essential Fatty Acids (EFA): are fatty acids that are required in the human diet. This means they cannot be synthesized by the body from other fatty acids and must be obtained from food. There are two closely related families of EFAs: ω-3 (or omega-3 or n-3) and ω-6 (omega-6, n-6.) They were originally designated as vitamin F when they were discovered as essential nutrients in 1923. Around 1930, it was realized that they are better classified with the fats than with the vitamins. Essential fatty acids play a part in many metabolic processes, and there is evidence to suggest that low levels of essential fatty acids, or the wrong balance of types among the essential fatty acids, may be a factor in a number of illnesses. Some of the food sources of ω-3 and ω-6 fatty acids are fish and shellfish, flaxseed (linseed), soya oil, canola (rapeseed) oil, hemp oil, chia seeds, pumpkin seeds, sunflower seeds, leafy vegetables and walnuts.

Epigallocatechin-3-Gallate (EGCG): This is the polyphenol most strongly associated with cancer prevention found in green and black tea.

Ellagic Acid: Has powerful antioxidant, anti-mutagen and anti-cancer properties. Studies have shown the anti-cancer activity on cancer cells of the breast, esophagus, skin, colon, prostate and pancreas. It can bind with cancer causing molecules, making them inactive and is chemoprotective against various chemically induced cancers. Ellagic acid helps eliminate excess nickel from the body. Plants produce ellagic acid to protect themselves from microbiological infection and pests. Its present in many red fruits and berries, including raspberries, strawberries, blackberries, cranberries, apples and pomegranate and some nuts including pecans and walnuts. The highest levels of ellagic acid are found in raspberries.

Eicosapentaenoic Acid (EPA): This is found in fish oils of cod liver, herring, mackerel, salmon, menhaden and sardines. It is also found in human breast milk. The body has a limited ability to manufacture EPA by converting the essential fatty acid, alpha-linolenic acid (ALA) which is found in flaxseed oil, canola oil or walnuts. Most fish oil supplements are 18% EPA and 12% DHA, or a total of 30% omega-3. EPA helps keep blood triglycerides in check (high triglycerides are generally linked with increased risk of heart disease) and may inhibit the progression of atherosclerosis. EPA and DHA keep blood from clotting too quickly.

Epidemiological: This is the study of the distribution of diseases in populations and of factors that influence the occurrence of disease.

Equisetum Arvense (Horsetail): These are vascular plants, comprising 15 species of plants. Horsetail, an herbal remedy dating back to at least ancient Roman and Greek medicine, was used traditionally to stop bleeding, heal ulcers and wounds, and treat tuberculosis and kidney problems. Today, horsetail continues to have medicinal value. The plant's stems are rich in silica and silicic acids, which help mend broken bones and form collagen, an important protein found in connective tissue, skin, bone, cartilage and ligaments. Horsetail is also used to treat infections of the urinary tract, kidney and bladder stones, and as topical therapy for burns and wounds.

Fats (lipids): Lipid is a catch-all phrase for a wide variety of hydrocarbon-based molecules of biological origin that are predominantly non-polar or hydrophobic ("water-fearing"), meaning that they do not interact well with water. The function of lipids in the body include cell membrane structure, controls membrane fluidity, controls the flow of material in and out of cells, energy storage (for instance, fats stored in adipose tissue), mediate communication between cells, function in the transmission of information in cells and are required for metabolism, usually as coenzymes.

Flavoneglycosides: These are found in ginkgo biloba, their antioxidant properties are thought to help prevent damage to the cells in the brain by chemicals called free radicals.

Flavonoids: Known as bioflavonoids are antioxidants that prevent cancer-causing hormones from attaching to body cells. They protect the eyes and nerves and help with symptoms of allergies, arthritis and asthma. There are over 4,000 types, some well-known foods which contain flavonoids are citrus fruits, berries, apples, tea, carrots, peppers, cabbage, tomato, squash, eggplant, broccoli, cucumbers, onions, parsley, soybeans and soy products.

Folic Acid (folate): Forms of a water-soluble B vitamin. These occur naturally in food and can also be taken as supplements. Folate gets its name from the Latin word *folium*, leaf. Folate is necessary for the production and maintenance of new cells. This is especially important during periods of rapid cell division and growth such as infancy and pregnancy. Folate is needed to replicate DNA. It also helps prevent changes to DNA that may lead to cancer. Thus folate deficiency hinders DNA synthesis and cell division, affecting most clinically the bone marrow, a site of rapid cell turnover. Both adults and children need folate to make normal red blood cells and prevent anemia.

Free Radicals: Free radicals play an important role in a number of biological processes, some of which are necessary for life, such as the intracellular killing of bacteria and are implicated in certain cell signaling processes. The two most important oxygen-centered free radicals are superoxide and hydroxyl radical. They are derived from molecular oxygen under reducing conditions. However, because of their reactivity, these same free radicals can participate in unwanted side reactions resulting in cell damage. Many forms of cancer are thought to be the result of reactions between free radicals and DNA, resulting in mutations that can adversely affect the cell cycle and potentially lead to malignancy. Some of the symptoms of aging such as atherosclerosis are also attributed to free-radicals. In addition free radicals contribute to alcohol-induced liver damage, perhaps more than alcohol itself. Because free radicals are necessary for life, the body has a number of mechanisms to minimize free radical induced damage and to repair damage which does occur, such as the enzymes superoxide dismutase, catalase, glutathione peroxidase and glutathione reductase. In addition, antioxidants play a key role in these defense mechanisms.

Gamma-Tocopherol: Natural vitamin E exists in eight different forms or isomers, four tocopherols and four tocotrienols, alpha, beta, gamma and delta form are found in both the tocopherols and tocotrienols. Alpha-tocopherol and gamma-tocopherol are the two major forms of vitamin E found in human plasma and tissues. The dietary intake of gamma-tocopherol is at least two times that of alpha-tocopherol in Western diets. The results of a 1997 study suggest that the mixed forms of vitamin E found in food may be more beneficial than the alpha tocopherol form which is the main ingredient in supplements. About 75 per cent of the vitamin E found in food is the gamma tocopherol form while supplements may not contain any gamma tocopherol and it is possible that taking very high doses of alpha tocopherol may displace gamma tocopherol.

215

Gastric Adenocarcinomas: Stomach cancer

Glutathione: A sulfur-containing amino acid that is an important part of the body's antioxidant defense system. It boosts the structure of body proteins and assists in the transport of amino acids across cell membranes. The phytochemical limonene may boost the body's synthesis of a glutathione-containing enzyme that has antioxidant properties and helps to detoxify heavy metals and chemicals. Limonene is found in citrus fruit peels, cherries, green foods, soy products, and wheat. Several foods contain naturally occurring glutathione, (cooking destroys all glutathione in these foods) including avocado, watermelon, tomatoes, asparagus, grapefruit, apple, carrots and spinach. Optimal amounts of glutathione are necessary for supporting the immune system; it also helps the liver to detoxify chemicals, such as acetaminophen (active ingredient in pain relief medication), copper, and cadmium.

Glycemic Index (gi): An indicator of the ability of different types of foods that contain carbohydrate to raise the blood glucose levels within two hours. Foods containing carbohydrates that break down most quickly during digestion have the highest glycemic index. Also called the dietary glycemic index.

Glycogen: As the storage form of glucose, it's used by the body for energy when needed. It's stored in the liver and muscle. It's found in carbohydrates, natural sugars (fruit, vegetables, milk) and complex carbohydrates (grains, cereals, pasta) are the best choices.

Glucose: A simple sugar that is a major source of energy in the body. All carbohydrates are broken down into simple sugars and transported as glucose in the bloodstream. Carbohydrates are found in fruits, vegetables, grains and dairy products.

HMG Co-A Reductase: An important cellular metabolic pathway present in virtually all organisms, it produces cholesterol and various other biomolecules. Drugs which inhibit HMG-CoA reductase, known collectively as HMG-CoA reductase inhibitors (or "statins"), are used to lower serum cholesterol as a means of reducing the risk for cardiovascular disease. These drugs include atorvastatin (Lipitor), pravastatin (Pravachol), and simvastatin (Zocor).

Homocysteine: An amino acid produced by the body, usually as a byproduct of consuming meat. Homocysteine can damage blood vessels in several ways, injuring the cells that line arteries and stimulating the growth of smooth muscle cells. It can also disrupt normal blood clotting mechanisms, increasing the risk of clots that can bring on a heart attack or stroke. The ways to bring down homocysteine are by eating less meat and by taking supplements of the B vitamins folic acid (folate), B6 and B12 that are needed by the enzymes that process homocysteine.

Hydroxytyrosol: A phytochemical from olives and olive oil, it has similar antioxidant properties as alpha tocopherol found in Vitamin E.

Hypothyroidism: The disease state caused by insufficient production of thyroid hormone by the thyroid gland. Clinically apparent hypothyroidism usually warrants treatment. In case the hypothyroidism is due to dietary minerals and iodine, supplementation with these may prevent the need for hormonal treatment, but only if iodine deficiency has been documented, which is very rare in the Western world due to high salt intake.

Indoles: Help stimulate the production of detoxifying enzymes, attach to chemical carcinogens making them harmless, protect against cancer and increase the body's detoxification functions. Foods containing indoles are cabbage, cauliflower, broccoli, Brussels sprouts, kale, collard greens, mustard greens and turnips.

Interferon: A class of natural proteins produced by the cells of the immune systems of most animals in response to challenges by foreign agents such as viruses, bacteria, parasites and tumor cells.

Interleukin 2: An interleukin, or hormone of the immune system that is instrumental in the body's natural response to microbial infection and in discriminating between foreign (nonself) and self.

Inulin: Used by some plants as a means of storing energy and is typically found in roots or rhizomes. It's used increasingly in foods, because it has excellent nutritional and functional characteristics, it increases calcium absorption and possibly magnesium absorption, while promoting probiotic bacteria. It has a minimal impact on blood sugar, making it suitable for diabetics and potentially helpful in managing blood sugar-related illnesses.

Ischemic Stroke: Due to a blood clot cutting off flow in a cerebral artery (the brain)

Isoflavones: Polyphenolic compounds produced almost exclusively by the members of the bean-family. They are long known for their estrogen-like effect on mammals. They are also very strong antioxidants. Various legumes including kudzu, lupine, fava bean, and soy contained substantial amounts of isoflavones. Highly processed foods made from legumes, such as tofu, retained most of their isoflavone content, with the exception of fermented miso, which actually had increased levels. Other dietary sources include chick pea, alfalfa sprouts and peanuts.

International Units (IU): A unit of measurement for the amount of a substance, based on measured biological activity (or effect). The precise definition of one IU differs from substance to substance and is established by international agreement.

L-Carnitine: Known as carnitine, is a quaternary ammonium compound derived from the amino acid lysine or methionine and is responsible for the transport of fatty acids into the mitochondria. It's chemically similar to Choline and is manufactured within the body in the liver and kidneys. The best source of natural carnitine is in red meat, seafood, dairy products and avocado. It is often sold as a nutritional supplement. Originally found as a growth factor for mealworms, vitamin C (ascorbic acid) is essential to the synthesis of carnitine. L-Carnitine is the main form of carnitine synthesized within the human body. It is 100% pure carnitine and is a common form found in supplements.

L-Ergothioneine: A powerful antioxidant, found in mushrooms. Shiitake, oyster, king oyster and maitake mushrooms contain the highest amounts of ergothioneine, with up to 13 mg in a 3-ounce serving. This equals forty times as much as is found in wheat germ. Of the most commonly consumed mushrooms, portobellas and criminis have the most L-ergothioneine, followed by white buttons. L-ergothionene is not destroyed when mushrooms are cooked.

Lactobacteria: Are the friendly bacteria that reside in your colon. Their job is to assist with end result digestion and keep harmful bacteria at bay. When your friendly lactobacteria are doing their job, (a) your colon maintains an acid environment, (b) harmful bacteria are kept in check, and (c) bowel movements can become effortless and nearly odorless

L-Taurine: Although it is often called an amino acid, it is not, it's an acidic chemical substance found in high abundance in the tissues of fish and meats. It's manufactured endogenously within the liver from cysteine and methionine. Some conditions that taurine might be useful in treating include: cardiovascular diseases, hypercholesterolemia, epilepsy and other seizure disorders, macular degeneration, Alzheimer's disease, liver disorders, alcoholism, and cystic fibrosis. Recent studies show that taurine supplements taken by mice on a high-fat diet reduced their overall weight. Studies have yet to be done on the effect of taurine on obesity in humans. Taurine can cure nervous tics/twitches around one's eyes, which was long thought to be incurable.

Lecithin: Is needed by every cell in the body and is a key building block of cell membranes; without it, they would harden. Lecithin protects cells from oxidation and largely comprises the protective sheaths surrounding the brain. More recently, lecithin has been proposed as a remedy for various psychological and neurological diseases, such as Tourette's syndrome, Alzheimer's disease, and bipolar disorder (also known as manic depression). It contains a substance called phosphatidylcholine (PC) that is presumed to be responsible for its medicinal effects. Phosphatidylcholine is a major part of the membranes surrounding our cells. However, when you consume phosphatidylcholine it is broken down into the nutrient choline rather than being carried directly to cell membranes. Choline acts like folate, TMG (trimethylglycine), and SAMe to promote methylation. It is also used to make acetylcholine, a nerve chemical essential for proper brain function.

Lentinan: Comes from the shitake mushroom. Lentinan's active polysaccharide 1,3 beta glucan is not cytotoxic but seems to enhance T-helper cell function, increase stimulation of interleukin, interferon, and normal killer cells. In addition to antitumor activity, it also possesses immune-regulatory effects, anti-viral activity, antimicrobial properties and cholesterol-lowering effects

Lipids: *see fats*

Lutein: An antioxidant known to reduce the risk of macular degeneration—an eye disease eventually causing blindness—and is thought to protect against cancer. Foods that contain lutein are kale, chard, spinach, turnip greens, chicory, radicchio, arugula, mustard greens and dandelion.

Lycopene: A subgroup of carotenoids, lycopene antioxidants have been found to lower the risk of prostate, breast, lung, gastrointestinal, cervical, bladder and endometrial cancer cells. Foods containing lycopene are cooked tomatoes, pink or red grapefruit, watermelon, guava and persimmons.

Lymphokines: Are produced by T cells, direct the immune system response by signaling between its cells. Lymphokines attract macrophages to the infected site and prepare them to attack the invaders.

Macrophages: Macrophages role is to engulf and then digest cellular debris and pathogens either as stationary or mobile cells, and to stimulate lymphocytes and other immune cells to respond to the pathogen. Macrophages are unable to divide and must mature from monocytes produced in the bone marrow.

Metastasis: Is the spread of cancer from its primary site to other places in the body.

Mitochondria: Is the site of the cell's energy production. The number of mitochondrion in each cell varies according to the individual energy requirements for that cell. Cardiac muscles contain thousands of mitochondrion per cell while some other types of cells only contain dozens (the average number of mitochondrion in a human cell is 1,000).

Monosaccharides: The simplest form of carbohydrates (sugar). They consist of one sugar and are usually colorless, water-soluble, crystalline solids. Some monosaccharides have a sweet taste. Examples of monosaccharides include glucose (dextrose), fructose, galactose and ribose.

Monosodium Glutamate (MSG): A sodium salt of glutamic acid. MSG is a food additive. There have been numerous studies of allergies and/or sensitivities to MSG, attributed to the free glutamic acid component, which has been blamed for causing a wide variety of physical symptoms such as migraines, nausea, digestive upsets, drowsiness, heart palpitations, hair loss, asthma, anaphylactic shock, rapidly increasing diabetes, and many other complaints. MSG may also be present in a wide variety of other additives, including hydrolyzed vegetable proteins, hydrolyzed yeast, and hydrolyzed soy extracts. MSG is known to be more toxic than Glutamic Acid, this is due to MSG being more readily absorbed by the body compared to Glutamic Acid. The increased toxicity of MSG is also believed to occur from the presence of the D-Glutamic Acid form of Glutamic Acid (as opposed to L-Glutamic Acid).

Myelin Sheaths: The cover that surrounds many nerve cells and helps to increase the speed by which information travels along the nerve.

Net Carbohydrates: A term developed by manufacturers to describe the carbohydrates that have a significant impact on blood sugar levels. While there is no regulatory definition of this term, it is generally calculated by subtracting the grams of "dietary fiber" from the "total carbohydrates" on the nutrition label. Although dietary fiber is a carbohydrate, it can't be broken down into sugar molecules, and so passes through the body mostly undigested.

Nutrients: Proteins, carbohydrates, fats, vitamins and minerals provided by food and necessary for growth and the maintenance of life.

Nitric Oxide: In the body, nitric oxide is involved in oxygen transport to the tissues, the transmission of nerve impulses, and other physiological activities. Nitric oxide is now thought to play a role in blood pressure regulation, control of blood clotting, immune defense, digestion, the senses of sight and smell, and possibly learning and memory. Nitric oxide may also participate in disease processes such as diabetes, stroke, hypertension, impotence, septic shock, and long-term depression.

Oleuropein: A highly bitter, naturally occurring chemical that renders the unprocessed olive inedible raw or even cooked, unlike any other fruit. Olives intended for eating must have the oleuropein removed by a curing process. Oleuropein is also found in the leaves of the olive tree, is a powerful antioxidant and used as an antimicrobial and antifungal supplement. It's also been found to help reduce LDL cholesterol levels.

Omega-3: Any of several polyunsaturated fatty acids found in leafy green vegetables, vegetable oils, and fish such as salmon and mackerel, capable of reducing serum cholesterol levels and having anticoagulant properties. Key omega-3 fatty acids include eicosapentaenoic acid (EPA) and docosahexanoic acid (DHA), both found primarily in oily cold-water fish such as tuna, salmon, and mackerel. Aside from fresh seaweed, a staple of many cultures, plant foods rarely contain EPA or DHA. However, a third omega-3, called alpha-linolenic acid (ALA), is found primarily in dark green leafy vegetables, flaxseed oils, and certain vegetable oils. Although ALA has different effects on the body than EPA and DHA do, the body has enzymes that can convert ALA to EPA. All three are important to human health.

Omega-6: Some medical research has suggested that excessive levels of omega-6 acids, relative to omega-3 acids, may increase the probability of a number of diseases. Modern Western diets typically have ratios of omega-6 to omega-3 in excess of 10 to 1, some as high as 30 to 1. The optimal ratio is thought to be 4 to 1 or lower. The most healthful of the omega-6s are those that contain linoleic acid. These convert in the body to gamma linoleic acid (GLA) and ultimately to prostaglandins, hormone-like molecules that help regulate Inflammation and blood pressure as well as heart, gastrointestinal, and kidney functions. The healing powers of a number of therapeutic oils rich in omega-6–including evening primrose oil (EPO), borage oil, black currant seed oil, and flaxseed oil, can be attributed to their high concentrations of GLA.

Omega-9 (oleic acid): are a class of unsaturated fatty acids, some are common components of animal fat and vegetable oil. Oleic acid is a main component of olive oil and other monounsaturated fats. Omega-9 fatty acids are not classed as essential fatty acids (EFA). This is both because they can be created by the human body from unsaturated fat.

Oligomeric Proanthocyanidins (OPC's): A class of flavonoid complexes found in grape seeds and skin, and dark chocolate, that act as antioxidants. It's proanthocyanidins antioxidant activity plays a role in the stabilization of collagen and maintenance of elastin–two critical proteins in connective tissue that support organs, joints, blood vessels, and muscle. OPCs may help protect against the effects of internal and environmental stresses (that is, cigarette smoking, pollution, and supporting normal body metabolic processes). The effects are; depressing blood fat, emulating blood vessels, lowering blood pressure, preventing blood vessel scleroses, dropping blood viscidity and preventing thrombus formation (a type of platelet clot). Additionally, studies have shown that OPCs may prevent cardiovascular disease by counteracting the negative effects of high cholesterol on the heart and blood vessels.

Opioids: Considered stress hormones and are manufactured by the body to reduce stress and relieve pain.

Oxygen Radical Absorbance Capacity (ORAC): is a scalar value useful for comparing the antioxidant content of different foods or nutritional supplements.

Osteoarthritis: Known as degenerative arthritis or degenerative joint disease is a condition in which low-grade inflammation results in pain in the joints, caused by wearing of the cartilage that covers and acts as a cushion inside joints.

Osteoblasts: Act on compact bone to store calcium in the matrix. This activity is controlled by hormones calcitonin and parathyroid hormone secreted by the thyroid and parathyroid endocrine glands. Bone is constantly being reshaped by osteoblasts, which build bone, and osteoclasts, which resorb bone.

Osteoclasts: They are involved in the natural turnover of bone tissue along with osteoblasts. Osteoclasts are regulated by several hormones, including parathyroid hormone (PTH) from the parathyroid gland, calcitonin from the thyroid gland, and growth factor interleukin 6 (IL-6). This last hormone, IL-6, is one of the factors in the disease osteoporosis, which is an imbalance between bone resorption and bone formation.

Osteopenia: A decrease in bone mineral density that can be a precursor condition to osteoporosis. However, not every person diagnosed with osteopenia will develop osteoporosis.

Osteoporotic Fractures: Compression fractures usually caused by osteoporosis in white women 50 years and older, the risk of osteoporotic fracture is nearly 40 percent over their remaining lifetime.

Oxidative Stress: A medical term for damage to animal or plant cells (and thereby the organs and tissues composed of those cells) caused by reactive oxygen species, which include (but are not limited to) superoxide, singlet oxygen, peroxynitrite or hydrogen peroxide. It is defined as an imbalance between pro-oxidants and anti-oxidants, with the former prevailing.

Phenylethyl Isothiocyanate (PEITC): is a promising chemoprotective compound. It may inhibit the ability of the primary carcinogenic substance in tobacco (4-(methylnitrosamino)-1-(3-pyridyl-1-butanone)) that is the underlying cause of tobacco-induced lung cancer. Watercress is the richest natural source of a compound called PEITC, which gives the plant its unique peppery flavor and in a wide number of scientific studies has been shown to have powerful anti cancer properties.

Phagocytic: In animals, phagocytosis is performed by specialized cells called phagocytes, which serve to remove foreign bodies and thus fight infection. The most important facet of phagocytosis is its control of inflammation.

Phenylalanine: An essential amino acid. It exists in two forms, a *D* and an *L* form, which are mirror-image molecules of each other. *L*-phenylalanine can also be converted into *L*-tyrosine, another one of the twenty protein-forming amino acids. *L*-tyrosine is converted into L-DOPA, which is further converted into dopamine, norepinephrine, and epinephrine. *D*-phenylalanine can be converted only into phenylethylamine. The synthesized mix DL-Phenylalanine (DLPA), which is a combination of the D- and L- forms is used as a nutritional supplement. Research indicates that DLPA can be an effective part of an overall program to fight chronic pain and depression in some cases, including the mood swings of premenstrual syndrome (PMS). Some sources contend that DLPA can increase energy and mental alertness, as well as heighten the ability to focus in individuals with attention deficit hyperactivity disorder (ADHD).

Phosphatidylcholine: Phosphatidylcholine (once given the name "lecithin") is usually the most abundant phospholipid in animal and plants, often amounting to almost 50% of the total. It is the key building block of membrane bilayers. Phosphatidylcholine is also the principal phospholipid circulating in plasma, where it is an integral component of the lipoproteins, especially the HDL. It protects cells from oxidation and largely comprises the protective sheaths sur-rounding the brain.

Phytochemicals (phytonutrients): In broad terms, they are said to be any chemical or nutrient derived from a plant source. They are usually used to refer to compounds found in plants that are not required for normal functioning of the body but that nonetheless have a beneficial effect on health. Phytochemicals naturally occur in vegetables and fruit.

Phytonutrients: *see phytochemicals*

Phytosterol: The term Phytosterols refers to any sterol or stanol derived from plants. More than 40 types of phytosterols have been identified to date. As early as 1951, it was shown that phytosterols lowered cholesterol in chickens, and subsequently they were found to lower cholesterol in humans by inhibiting the absorption of cholesterol in the diet. Food sources include rice bran oil, avocado, alfalfa sprouts, olives and olive oil, figs, barley, oats, wheat and fennel.

Polyphenol: The most abundant group of plant phenolic compounds, known to provide much of the flavor, color, and taste to fruits, vegetables, seeds, and other parts of the plants. As dietary sources of biologically active compounds they prove to be valuable for health. They have been linked to reduce the risk of cardiovascular disease, cancer, and other degenerative diseases. The various health benefits of polyphenols have been associated with their antioxidant, antibacterial, anti-inflammatory, and anti-allergenic properties.

Polysaccharides (*glycans*): Any class of carbohydrates, such as starch and cellulose, consisting of a number of monosaccharides joined by glycosidic bonds.

Polyunsaturates: An omega-6 fatty acid, the "healthy fat," recommended daily consumption is between 5% and 10%. Omega-6 and omega-3 fatty acids compete with each other for absorption; it's recommended to consume equal amounts of each for optimal health. Sources for omega-6 are evening primrose oil, borage seed oil, black current oil, grape seed oil, walnut oil, safflower oil, pine nuts, peanuts and avocado. Also found in fish and seafood (herring, salmon, mackerel, halibut).

Prebiotic: Food substances which promote the growth of beneficial bacteria in the intestines.

Proanthocyanidins: Powerful antioxidants found in chocolate, green tea and red wine.

Probiotic: Bacterial cultures are intended to assist the body's naturally occurring flora within the digestive tract to reestablish themselves. The body contains a miniature ecology of microbes, collectively known as the gut flora. The number of bacterial types can be thrown out of balance by a wide range of circumstances including the use of antibiotics or other drugs, excess alcohol, stress, disease, exposure to toxic substances, or even the use of antibacterial soap. In cases like these, the bacteria that work well with our bodies may decrease in number, an event which allows harmful competitors to thrive, to the detriment of our health.

Proteoglycans: A major component of the animal extracellular matrix (collagen), the "filler" substance existing between cells in an organism. They're distributed almost everywhere in the body. Their size and structure vary. The basic structure of all proteoglycans includes a core protein and at least one, but frequently more (up to tens or hundreds) carbohydrate chains, so called glycosaminoglycans.

Pterostilbene: An antioxidant compound that is found in colorful fruit, especially blueberries and cranberries. Like resveratrol, a compound which has been identified in grapes and red wines, pterostilbene belongs to a group of compounds called phytoalexins which are produced by plants in response to stresses such as fungal infections and ultraviolet light. Pterostilbene is known to help regulate blood sugar and may help fight type-2 diabetes.

Quercetin: This is found to be the most active of the flavonoids in studies, and many medicinal plants owe much of their activity to their high quercetin content. It has demonstrated significant anti-inflammatory activity because of direct inhibition of several initial processes of inflammation. Also quercetin shows remarkable anti-tumour properties.

Resveratrol: A class of polyphenol compounds produced as a part of a plant's defense system against disease. It's produced (in the plants in which it is present) during times of environmental stress, such as adverse weather, insect attack, animal attack or pathogenic attack. It is both water-soluble and fat-soluble. It inhibits tumor formation and breaks down "bad," LDL cholesterol; lowers risk of atherosclerosis. Found in grapes (particularly red) and wine, as well as peanuts, cranberries and mulberries.

Recommended Dietary Allowances (RDA): Nutrient intake recommendations from the Institute of Medicine, an arm of the American Academy of Sciences. RDAs are safe levels of intake for essential nutrients, based on current scientific knowledge. They are set to meet the known nutrient needs of practically all healthy people. RDAs have been around and updated regularly for more than 50 years. RDAs are gradually being replaced by revised guidelines called Dietary Reference Intakes or DRIs.

Saturated Fat: Shown to raise cholesterol, associated with a risk of heart disease. Found in butter, lard, meat, poultry, whole-milk dairy foods, palm oil and coconut oil.

S-Adenosylmethionine (SAMe): An enzymatic cofactor involved in methyl group transfers. It helps in the maintenance of the action of several hormones and neurotransmitters that affect mood. SAMe has been shown to have a therapeutic effect in liver disease, mood disorders and osteoporosis, many of which are supported by hundreds of research articles.

Sebum: The sebaceous glands in the skin of mammals secrete an oily substance called sebum that is made of fat (lipids) and the debris of dead fat-producing cells.

Selenium: Selenium is an essential micronutrient in all known forms of life. In humans, selenium is a trace element nutrient which functions as cofactor for reduction of antioxidant enzymes such as glutathione peroxidases. It also plays a role in the functioning of the thyroid gland by participating as a cofactor for thyroid hormone. RDA: 55 mg for women and 70 mg for men.

Serotonin: This is believed to play an important role in the regulation of mood, sleep, emesis (vomiting), sexuality and appetite. Serotonin is an inhibitory neurotransmitter. Men generally have far higher (brain) serotonin levels than women. Recent research suggests that serotonin also plays an important role in liver regeneration and induces cell division throughout the body. The amino acid tryptophan and its metabolite 5-hydroxytryptophan (5-HTP), from which serotonin is synthesized, crosses the blood-brain barrier. These agents are available as dietary supplements and may be effective serotonergic agents. Intense exercise may increase brain serotonin levels.

Superoxide Dismutase (SOD): An important antioxidant defense in nearly all cells exposed to oxygen. The presence of SOD has been shown to help protect many types of cells from the free radical damage that is important in aging, and ischemic tissue damage. SOD also helps protect cells from DNA damage, lipid peroxidation, ionizing radiation damage, protein denaturation, and many other forms of progressive cell degradation.

Spirulina (blue green algae): is a nutrient dense Superfood cultivated as a food source in many parts of the world. It is a powerful antioxidant, and known to help detoxify mercury and lead from the body. Records of the Spanish Conquistadores suggest the Aztecs may have harvested Spirulina for use as a food.

Sulforaphane: Are cancer inhibitors and also enhance detoxification. Foods containing sulforaphane are broccoli, cauliflower, Brussels sprouts, kale and turnips.

Syndrome X (Metabolic syndrome): A combination of medical disorders that affect a large number of people in a clustered fashion. In some studies, the prevalence in the USA is calculated as being up to 25% of the population, the end result of which increases risks for cardiovascular disease and diabetes. The causes of metabolic syndrome are extremely complex. Most patients are older, obese and have a degree of insulin resistance. There is debate regarding whether obesity or insulin resistance is the cause of the metabolic syndrome or a byproduct of a more far-reaching metabolic derangement. Systemic inflammation: a number of inflammatory markers are often increased.

Synovial Fluid: Reduces friction between the articular cartilage and other tissues in joints to lubricate and cushion them during movement.

Terpenoids: Any compound with an isoprenoid structure similar to that of the terpene hydrocarbons found in plants.

Tocopherols: *see gamma tocopherols*

Tryptophan: An amino acid and essential in human nutrition. Tryptophan is a precursor for serotonin (a neurotransmitter), melatonin (a neurohormone), and niacin.

Tyrosine: Converted to DOPA by tyrosine hydroxylase, an enzyme. It plays a key role in signal transduction, it is also a precursor to the thyroid hormones thyroxine and triiodothyronine, the pigment melanin, and the biologically-active dopamine, norepinephrine and epinephrine.

Zeaxanthin: One of the two carotenoids contained within the retina. There is epidemiological evidence of a relationship between low plasma concentrations of lutein and zeaxanthin on the one hand, and the risk of developing age-related macular degeneration (AMD) on the other. Some studies support the view that supplemental lutein and/or zeaxanthin help protect against AMD. There is also epidemiological evidence that increasing lutein and zeaxanthin intake lowers the risk of cataract development.

Nutritional Dictionary

. . . .

Vitamin A *(a.k.a. pre-formed Retinol;Beta-Carotene)*

What it's good for: Promotes growth and repair of body tissue, healthy eyes, good night vision and a strong immune system.

Where you get it: Liver and fish oils, whole and fortified milk and eggs. Carrots, sweet potatoes, spinach and other leafy green veggies, yellow squash, apples and apricots provide Beta and other carotenes.

RDA: 10,000 IU for adult women and men.

Vitamin B-1 *(a.k.a. Thiamine)*

What it's good for: Helps convert food into energy, nerve functions, growth and muscle tone.

Where you get it: Wheat germ, pork, whole and enriched grains, dried beans, seeds and nuts.

RDA: Between 1.1 to 1.5 mg for adults.

Vitamin B-2 *(a.k.a. Riboflavin)*

What it's good for: Releases energy, keeps red blood cells healthy, and makes hormones.

Where you get it: Dairy products, meats, poultry, whole and enriched grains, and green vegetables such as broccoli, turnip greens, aspargus and spinach.

Quick Tip: High doses of B-2 may help prevent migraine headaches.

RDA: Between 1.3 to 1.7 mg for adults.

Vitamin B-3 *(a.k.a Niacin)*

What it's good for: Releases energy, important for a healthy digestive system, blood circulation, nerve function, and appetite.

Where you get it: Poultry, fish, whole and enriched grains, dried beans and peas.

RDA: Between 15 to 19 mg for adults.

Vitamin B-5 *(a.k.a Pantothenic Acid)*

What it's good for: Converts food into energy, necessary to make important hormones, vitamin D and red blood cells.

Where you get it: Found in almost all foods.

RDA: None.

Vitamin B-6 *(a.k.a Pyridoxine)*

What it's good for: Helps convert food into energy, keeps red blood cells healthy, makes antibodies, maintains nerve function, enhances the immune system, and helps prevent heart disease.

Where you get it: Poultry, fish, pork, eggs, and whole grains.

Quick Tip: Small doses of B-6 may help alleviate morning sickness. Check with your doctor.

RDA: Between 1.6 to 2.0 mg for adults.

Quick Tip 2: B-6 in high doses can cause balance difficulties, and nerve injury.

Vitamin B-12 *(a.k.a. Cobalamin)*

What it's good for: Releases energy from food, keeps red blood cells healthy, helps maintain the nervous system, boosts the immune system, and helps prevent heart disease.

Where you get it: Dairy products, lean beef, fish, poultry and eggs.

RDA: 2 mcg for adults.

Biotin

What it's good for: Metabolizes fats, proteins and carbohydrates, helps in the transfer of carbon dioxide and assists in various metabolic chemical conversions.

Where you get it: Cheese, beef liver, cauliflower, eggs, mushrooms, chicken breast, salmon and spinach.

Suggested Daily Value: 300 mcg for adults.

Vitamin C

What it's good for: Helps wounds heal, strengthens blood vessels, builds connective tissue, healthy gums, skin and promotes strong teeth and bones. May boost immunity.

Where you get it: Citrus fruits, strawberries, green and red peppers, collard and mustard greens, broccoli, spinach, tomatoes, potatoes, kiwi, guava and parsley.

RDA: 75 mg for women, 90 mg for men.

Calcium

What it's good for: Supports bones, teeth, muscle tissue, regulates the heartbeat, muscle action, nerve function, and blood clotting.

Where you get it: Dairy products, calcium-fortified orange juice or soy milk, salmon with bones, and green leafy vegetables such as broccoli, kale, and collards.

RDA: 1,000 mg for adults.

Chromium

What it's good for: Acts cooperatively with other substances to control insulin and certain enzymes.

Where you get it: Cheese, whole grains, meat, peas, beans and blackstrap molasses.

RDA: None.

Copper

What it's good for: Formation of red blood cells, pigment, and bone health.

Where you get it: Nuts, black pepper, blackstrap molasses and cocoa.

RDA: None.

Vitamin D

What it's good for: Calcium and phosphorus metabolism, aids bone growth and integrity, and promotes strong teeth.

Where you get it: Fortified milk, egg yolks and fatty fish, like herring, kipper and mackerel.

RDA: 5-10 mcg for adults.

Vitamin E

What it's good for: Antioxidant powers protect cell membranes, essential for red blood cells, aids cellular respiration and protects lung tissue from pollution.

Where you get it: Vegetable oils, wheat germ, green leafy vegetables, seeds, nuts, seafood, apples, carrots and celery.

RDA: 15 mg alpha-tocopherol for adults.

Fiber

What it's good for: Lowers cholesterol and blood sugar levels, helps move waste through the intestines. Diets rich in plant fiber are related to a reduction of heart disease, colon cancer and diabetes.

Where you get it: Fruits, vegetables and whole-grains.

Quick Tip: If you're increasing your fiber intake, do it slowly to avoid stomach upset. Also, drink lots of water.

RDA: None.

Folate

What it's good for: Helps cells grow and divide, reduces risk of certain birth defects, important for red blood cells and crucial in creating amino acids.

Where you get it: Green leafy vegetables, dried beans, liver, poultry, fortified cereals, oranges and nuts.

Quick Tip: Pregnant women or women trying to conceive are often told to take folate.

RDA: 400 mcg for adults.

Iodine

What it's good for: Making thyroid hormones that control metabolism.

Where you get it: Lobster, shrimp, milk, iodized salt and sea vegetables.

RDA: 150 mcg for adults.

Iron

What it's good for: Making hemoglobin in blood and myoglobin in muscle, which supply oxygen to cells.

Where you get it: Rice bran, wheat bran, fish, liver, molasses, kelp, cocoa, and spirulina.

RDA: Between 10 to 12 mg for men and 12 to 15 mg for women.

Quick Tip: Iron supplements even in small amounts can be toxic to young children.

Vitamin K

What it's good for: Helps blood clot and bone formation.

Where you get it: Turnip greens, alfalfa, kale, brussels sprouts, cabbage, spinach, parsley, and green tea.

RDA: Between 60 to 65 mcg for women and 70 to 80 mcg for men.

Magnesium

What it's good for: Enzyme activation, nerve and muscle function, and bone growth.

Where you get it: Nuts, meats, leafy vegetables, whole grains, beans and legumes.

Quick Tip: Inadequate magnesium intake frequently causes muscle spasms, and has been associated with caridovascular disease, diabetes, high blood pressure, anxiety disorders and osteoporosis.

RDA: Between 280 to 300 mg for women, 350 to 400 mg for men.

Manganese

What it's good for: Essential for reproductive function, physical growth, normal formation of bones and cartilage and normal brain function.

Where you get it: Whole grains and cereals, fruits, vegetables, tea, walnuts, pecans, Brazil nuts, and hops.

RDA: None.

Molybdenum

What it's good for: It plays a vital role in three important enzymes systems, uric acid formation, iron utilization, in carbohydrate metabolism and sulfite detoxifications.

Where you get it: Lentils, split peas, liver, cauliflower, spinach, green peas, and wheat germ.

RDA: None.

Phosphorus

What it's good for: Helps form bones and teeth, builds muscle and is involved in almost all metabolic actions in the body.

Where you get it: Milk, meat, poultry, fish, eggs, whole grains, seeds and nuts.

RDA: 800 mg to 1,200 mg for adults.

Potassium

What it's good for: Helps keep blood pressure down and aids muscle contractions, aids healthy electrical activity in the heart and rapid transmission of nerve impulses throughout the body.

Where you get it: Dried fruits, bananas, potatoes, most raw vegetables, citrus fruits, molasses, and pistachio nuts.

RDA: None.

Protein

What it's good for: Keeps the body running, made from different combinations of amino acids.

Where you get it: Meat, eggs, dairy products, beans, whole grains, and vegetables.

RDA: Between 46 and 63 g for adults.

Sodium

What it's good for: Regulates and balances the amount of fluids outside the cells in the body. Aids in muscle contractions and nerve function.

Where you get it: Processed foods and table salt.

RDA: None.

Zinc

What it's good for: Essential for normal growth, development and immunity. Helps maintain skin, hair and bones. Keeps reproductive organs functioning and helps in the perception of taste and the ability to see at night.

Where you get it: Brazil nuts, beef, poultry, liver, oysters, eggs and dairy products.

RDA: Between 12 to 15 mg for women and 15 mg for men.

Index